Date Due

BRODART, INC.   Cat. No. 23 233   Printed in U.S.A.

African-American Women's Health and Social Issues

AFRICAN-AMERICAN WOMEN'S HEALTH AND SOCIAL ISSUES

Edited by
Catherine Fisher Collins

Foreword by
Vivian W. Pinn

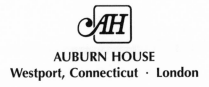

AUBURN HOUSE
Westport, Connecticut · London

Library of Congress Cataloging-in-Publication Data

African-American women's health and social issues / edited by
   Catherine Fisher Collins ; foreword by Vivian W. Pinn.
       p.   cm.
   Includes bibliographical references and index.
   ISBN 0–86569–250–5 (alk. paper)
       1. Afro-American women—Health and hygiene.   2. Afro-American
   women—Diseases.   3. Afro-American women—Social conditions.
   I. Collins, Catherine Fisher.
   RA448.5.N4A445   1996
   613'.04244'08996073—dc20   96–10376

British Library Cataloguing in Publication Data is available.

Library of Congress Catalog Card Number: 96–10376
ISBN: 0-86569-250-5

First published in 1996

Auburn House, 88 Post Road West, Westport, CT 06881
An imprint of Greenwood Publishing Group Inc.

Printed in the United States of America

The paper used in this book complies with the
Permanent Paper Standard issued by the National
Information Standards Organization (Z39.48-1984).

10 9 8 7 6 5 4 3 2 1

This book is dedicated to the late Herman Fisher Jr.
I love you and I miss you.

Your sister

Special love to the late Clyde A. Collins.

Your wife

Contents

Part II: Social Issues

Illustrations

FIGURES

Foreword

As African-American women, we can take great pride in the strength and solidarity that have sustained us and our community over many years. As Maya Angelou has so movingly described the African-American diaspora:

Although separated from our languages, our families and customs, we had dared to live. We had crossed the unknowable oceans in chains and had written its mystery into "Deep river, my home is over Jordan." Through the centuries of despair and dislocation, we had been creative, because we faced down death by daring to hope.[1]

Today, as the African-American community is threatened by disparate conditions that adversely affect our health and well-being, more than ever before, African-American women must draw upon the strength and character of their ancestors in facing down death by daring to hope—and by taking action to prevent the perpetuation of inequities and self-defeating behaviors.

Fortunately, our history from the time of Imhotep to the present is an impressive one and provides many guideposts for meeting the challenges that face us and our community. The same strength and solidarity that have sustained African-American women and their families throughout history can serve to sustain our community now and into the next millennium. Unfortunately, as African-American women we also share a long tradition of taking better care of others than of ourselves.

Overcoming the challenges to our individual and collective well-being demands appropriate action through the exercise of personal responsibility. But we must be mindful of the fact that focusing exclusively on the biologically based aspects of health is not enough. Physical and mental health and well-being are the by-products of an individual's culture, society, and familial and spiritual roots.

Fortunately, just as our lives at the end of the 20th century are being enriched through new roles and opportunities, so, too, is our ability to deal with the attendant stresses and pressures being enhanced by a new focus on the social, cultural, mental, and spiritual factors that influence health. Today, many of us recognize that the prescription for preserving good health may not necessarily be found in a medicine cabinet, but rather found within—in the same strength of spirit that has sustained African-American women for centuries.

The traditional definition of women's health was concerned almost exclusively with reproductive issues. By contrast, in the biomedical community today, study of women's health encompasses all the biological, familial, cultural, economic, emotional, psychological, and behavioral elements that coalesce to determine an individual woman's health over the course of her lifetime.

As Associate Director for Research on Women's Health at the National Institutes of Health (NIH), I enjoy the opportunity to redress inequities in prevention, detection, and treatment of illness among women of all races, cultures, and socioeconomic backgrounds, through biomedical and biobehavioral research on women's health at every stage of life, from childhood through the elderly years. Implicit in efforts to improve women's health is a tacit commitment to improving the health of all Americans, for women serve as caregivers to both the young and the elderly. Improving the health of women means improving the health of families and communities.

This book, *African-American Women's Health and Social Issues,* offers important insights concerning the health of African-American women. With its focus on addressing the biological, social, economic, and behavioral factors that contribute to our physical and mental health status, it enriches a growing body of literature on African-American women and provides a forum and opportunity to identify sources of strength and power within the African-American community that can be called upon in the effort to improve our individual and collective health. With hope, solidarity, knowledge, and commitment, we can overcome the forces that endanger our health and the health of the African-American community as a whole. This volume represents a significant step toward realizing that dream.

NOTE

1. Maya Angelou, *All God's Children Need Traveling Shoes* (New York: Random House, 1986).

Vivian W. Pinn, MD
Associate Director for Research on Women's Health
Director, Office of Research on Women's Health
National Institutes of Health

Acknowledgments

There are so many to thank, but I must first begin with the Almighty: thanks be to God, for all things are possible if you believe.

This book would not have been possible were it not for the "sisters" who made it possible. To each of the sisters/contributors—Peggy Brooks-Bertram, Reneé Daniel, Stacey Daniels, Cynthia Crawford-Green, Imani Lillie B. Fryar, Juanita K. Hunter, Jacqueline D. Skiller Jackson, Barbara A. Seals Nevergold, Dolores Davis-Penn, Noma L. Roberson, and E. Ginger Sullivan—your commitment to seeing this book to its fruition is far beyond a thank you. My wonderful parents, Catherine Lynch Fisher and the late Herman Fisher, Sr.—I love you. My daughter, Laura Harris, and son, Clyde II, you are the loves of my life; how do I thank you for being my children? Crystal and Kenneth II my beautiful grandchildren, you are so special—thank you. To Fay, my sister, and David, my brother, hugs and kisses. My colleagues at SUNY Empire State College, your many words of encouragement are important—thank you. To Professor Robert Heller, SUNY Buffalo, a special thank you for all your support. The technical assistance provided by Marvel Ross-Jones is, once again, beyond a thank you. Your smiles and never unnerving manner are a real inspiration; you are really a very special and spiritual person—God bless you. To the mothers in Jack and Jill of America, Inc. and sisters in the Links, Inc., thank you. And finally, to everyone I missed, know that you are all very special in my life and this book.

Introduction

This book's contributors are African-American women who are sensitive, caring, and knowledgeable about the health and social issues that plague their communities. For too many years the literature on these issues has been dominated by white male writers, followed by white females and black males, who all believe that they know what we want, when we know that the best authority about us, *is us*.

From this premise the deplorable health and social conditions that African-American women have to endure are explored from our authentic voices in 12 dynamic chapters. The book begins with a "Commentary on the Health and Social Status of African-American Women," which will help the reader to better understand the thrust of the chapters that follow.

In Part I, Health Issues, Chapter 1 presents AIDS, the worse pandemic to be unleashed on the African-American female. This disease, which is the leading cause of death for African-American women of childbearing age in the states of New York and New Jersey, where they comprise 72% of the population diagnosed with HIV/AIDS, is brought to the forefront from an Afrocentric perspective.

One of the most insidious diseases affecting the health of African-American women, lupus, is discussed in Chapter 2. Not only is this disease difficult to diagnose, there is a need to expand professional and public education about this disease that affects African-American women dispro-portionately. In this chapter the sociological and psychological aspects are presented in an effort to raise the consciousness of physicians of those women who may be experiencing vague neurological symptoms.

Addressing the issues of cancer, Chapter 3 will examine some of the important factors believed to be linked to the disproportionately high dis-ease rate among African-American females. Particularly of concern is the deplorable very low survival rate for low-income African-American female cancer patients.

Hypertension and its impact on the African-American community, with emphasis on the African-American female, will be explored in Chapter 4, from both cultural and medical management perspectives.

It is estimated that there are over 10 million Americans with some form of diabetes, the subject of Chapter 5. Many of these individuals are over-weight African-American women, where the disease is having the most devastating effects. With Type II diabetes (noninsulin dependent type) diet and exercise can effectively control it. Then why are there so many ampu-tations, strokes, and blindness among these women? This chapter will ad-dress some of the lifestyles, social constraints, and cultural influences that affect the outcomes for these women.

For too long African-American women have been too silent on the sub-ject of stress and alcohol abuse. We have seen the greatest increase in the abuse of alcohol among African-American women who are single parents and heads of household. Why? The "why" is addressed in Chapter 6 by looking at internal and external demands placed on African-American women and how needed resources have for some, but not all, been able to meet their demands. We must keep in mind that drinking is, for many, the pain relief sought from those social ills and daily assaults on women's very existence in various forms of discrimination, racism, and sexism of our times. With a nation that has failed to meet the basic human needs of its largest minority, can we really expect that the incidences of those condi-tions associated with this disease (cirrhosis, child abuse) will be eradi-cated?

Chapter 7 will discuss the status of research on the mental health of African-American women with emphasis on depression. It is further made clear why so many women of color suffer from depression.

In Part II, Social Issues that impact on African-American women are presented. The chapters contain subject matter that has not been thor-oughly explored from the African-American female perspective.

In Chapter 8 we are acquainted or reacquainted with the issues of homelessness. But the focus of this American shame is the African-Ameri-can women who are forced to live on the streets, many with small infants. Because women of color tend to have higher birth rates, single mothers and children jam the few homeless shelters. The issues that confront homeless women of color such as alcohol, substance abuse, family violence, and psychiatric/mental health problems are brought to our attention through the work completed on one of this nation's funded health programs for homeless women.

Most literature on the subject of Chapter 9, African-American elderly, is limited to the urban/inner-city dweller. In this chapter, the attitudes and knowledge about cancer prevention barriers experienced by the elderly will be addressed. The model developed from this research will help serve as a guide to intervention strategies to improve the health of elderly African-American female rural residents.

In recent years there has been a flurry of concern with white American adoption of minority children, as discussed in Chapter 10. The chapter will examine the issues related to transracial adoption, in particular to African-American children. The chapter will cite opposing arguments, but it clearly takes the position that transracial adoptions are not in the "best-interest" of the African-American child.

Chapter 11 will explore African-American women's reproductive rights, something that most groups tend to overlook when dealing with the issues. For too long women of color have been silent on the issues of reproductive rights. They have been exercising increasing control over their fertility, but this control is not without its ambivalence. Past attitudes, poor experience with health providers, and traditional beliefs about health and illness influence reproductive decisions made today. These and many other issues will be presented.

The central theme of Chapter 12 is those coping behaviors that help African-American women survive. There are cultural variations in how individuals handle oppression. Strategies appearing negative to the outside observer may be the appropriate mechanism for the oppressed to repossess or reconnect to cultural bearings. From the residual effects on the lives of the African slaves has evolved coping skills that African-Americans have incorporated into their lives. How successful these skills have been in shielding African-American women from the barrage of daily pressures will be presented through the works of others.

Commentary on the Health and Social Status of African-American Women

Catherine Fisher Collins

The health status of African-American women has received considerable attention over the last two decades, yet they remain the sickest of all American minorities and nonminorities. In this commentary I will present some of the health indicators that demonstrate the poor health status of African-American women, taking into account the impact of poverty, racism, sexism, poor education, limited or no access to health care services, and other related factors.

In seeking to understand how sick a population really is, one might investigate the life expectancy of that population. Often we are led to believe that African-American women, and other poor women, receive considerable health resources, driving up Medicaid health care costs. One might then expect their health status to be fairly good, if not excellent. In looking at one measurement—life expectancy, which "describes the likelihood of surviving to a given age at a given time in history" (Harper & Lambert, 1994, p. 16)—one might then assume that those who are supposedly using all of this health care would be in relatively good health.

Determining how long a person will live is based on age-specific death rates of the population at a certain time. Life expectancy is not only how long African-American women are expected to live, but it is also a good indication of how they are meeting the awesome challenges of society, as

Table 1
Life Expectancy of African-American and White Women, 1960–1992

Race	1960	1970	1980	1990	1992
White American	74.1	75.6	78.7	79.4	79.7
African American	66.3	68.3	72.5	73.6	73.9

Sources: For 1960, 1970 & 1980—Wegman (1990), Table 4, p. 841; for 1990 & 1992—
    Wegman (1993), Table 4, p. 747.

compared to other women. Unfortunately, the optimal health of a population is standardized by the healthiest in the country. Therefore, for this
commentary, white American women will be our comparative population.
The data in Table 1 indicate a very poor outlook for African-American
women.

Clearly these data indicate that the life expectancy of African-American
women has improved somewhat. However, the gains of white women in
42 years (5.6) when compared to the gains of African-American women
(7.6) appears to be less; but in reality, white women's life expectancy had
a much better start. In 1960 the life expectancy of white women was 74.1,
which is not on par with African-American women, whose life expectancy
was 66.3.

In an Urban League (Leffal, 1990) publication it was reported that African-American women have more undetected diseases and chronic and
acute illnesses than other women. Some of these illnesses may be due to
lifestyle behavior (e.g., cirrhosis of the liver) or genetics (glaucoma, sickle-
cell anemia), which may affect life expectancy. But in the context of poverty, racism, and sexism, access to health care survival is questionable. As
mentioned, poverty has an impact on health status. If you have money
you are usually educated and therefore can purchase health services from
providers whom you select and keep because they provide good care.

According to the Bureau of the Census (1992) there are 30 million African-Americans or 12.1% of the total population, and the largest minority
in America. It was also reported that of these 30 million, 16 million are
women, and poverty affected 35.5 percent of them in 1990. Furthermore,
48 percent of these women were heads of households with incomes below
the poverty level. Incomes that fall below the poverty level hamper pur-
chasing power for decent housing and nutritious food that is low in fat.
Inadequate access to the nearest free hospital clinics sets the stage for mal-
nutrition, lead poisoning, rat-infested housing, stress, and depression, leading to alcoholism and drug addiction. Each of these life-cry social and

economic experiences translates into exposure to certain illnesses (e.g., acquired immunodeficiency syndrome [AIDS]).

Furthermore, when poverty is facilitated by racism, disease states flourish. For example, in historical context of service delivery pre-1900s, meager health care was offered to free and sick female slaves. Their poor health condition led F. L. Hoffman (1897, p. 148) to state that blacks showed the least ability to compete in the struggle for existence, as justification to do nothing about the health needs of African Americans. As a result, African-American women, learned to endure many illnesses early on, dying at an alarming rate from childbirth and other preventable health conditions.

With limited access to hospital delivery rooms in the 1930s, some mothers survived. However, tuberculosis (TB) and syphilis held back any substantial gains, thus contributing to morbidity. Following the end of World War I, limited gains in health conditions were experienced by African-American women (Beardsley, 1990). The great depression served as the force that essentially eliminated some of the public health clinics and programs. It was not until the passage of the 1935 Social Security Act that some clinics in poor neighborhoods were reestablished. African-American women could then seek care in these free public health clinics and hospitals, created by the Hill Burton programs. Under Hill Burton, hospitals were more willing to allow African-American women to deliver in hospitals, once reserved only for white women, whether the bed was occupied or not. As more African-American women sought hospital care, it became very apparent that racism was not confined to their neighborhoods. A well-devised and -defined segregated health care delivery system developed, one for blacks and one for whites. This segregated health care system was challenged by the National Association for the Advancement of Colored People (NAACP), and the overt discrimination in health care became less distinguishable, because of potential loss of federal funding and the ability to sue under the Civil Rights Act of 1964. With better access to health care for African-American women, they still remain the sickest of American citizens.

The realization of having access is no guarantee that what you need is what you get. Furthermore, having insurance is no guarantee that the service you receive is equal to that provided for your white counterpart. Some 21% of African-Americans receive their health care from physicians in emergency rooms. Another 20% receive care from hospital clinics. When patients are treated with disrespect, it lowers their satisfaction with the care they have received, which may be a contributing factor to low follow-up visits. Moreover, access to health care by the 57% of African-Americans who are insured, and the 18% who have Medicaid, gives no guarantee that they will receive quality health care (Reed et al., 1993, p. 118). African-Americans are often reminded of the Tuskegee syphilis experiment and the recently reported wrong leg amputation of an African-American. With these and other historical accounts of the mistreatment of African-Americans, coupled with a racist provider, some would justify a skipped follow-up appointment or disregard a sore that will not heal.

If the lack of health insurance, access issues, racism, and poverty are not enough, lifestyle behaviors of African-American women seriously affect their health status. Sickness is often caused by inappropriate health habits and lifestyle behaviors, which make these women more susceptible to a variety of illnesses. Diseases such as diabetes mellitus predisposed by obesity, certain cancers (lung) related to smoking, cardiovascular diseases predisposed by high serum cholesterol, cirrhosis of the liver predisposed by alcohol consumption and drug addiction are all preventable yet each has devastating effects on the health status of African-American females.

In a study by the National Institute on Drug Abuse (NIDA) (1990) it was reported that black women are more likely than women of any other racial/ethnic group to have used crack cocaine. Black patients accounted for 39% (63,002) of the 160,170 drug-abuse-related emergency room visits, and for 30% of the 6,756 drug-abuse-related deaths reported by medical examiners. This included 41% of cocaine-related deaths and 31% of heroin/morphine-related deaths. As Donnie W. Watson, a clinical psychologist, states: "Some minority researchers see substance abuse as a secondary problem, resulting from individual responses to primary problems of oppression, racism, economic deprivation, stress, and despair in society" (Braithwaite & Taylor, 1992, p. 64).

The increase in the use of injectable, short-duration drugs, like cocaine, and the return to the streets of heroin use have provided an avenue for the spread of the AIDS virus. This increase is supported by data from *The Women's Health Data Book* (Horton, 1992 & 1995), which reports that in 1992 "the death rate for [human immunodeficiency virus (HIV)] infection for persons 25–44 years of age was 12 times higher for black women (38.0 per 100,000) than for white women (3.3 per 100,000)" (Horton, 1995, p. 47).

Through their drug-addicted behavior the health status of African-American women was further compromised and affected by exposure to a variety of sexually transmitted diseases (STDs), which occur in the general population at about 12 million cases per year (Horton, 1992, p. 27). Among these STDs, syphilis and gonorrhea are at epidemic proportions, as the following data as reported by (Horton, 1992, p. 28) suggest:

• Syphilis prevalence rates between 1985 and 1989 indicate that the rate for black women increased by 176% from 35.8 to 98.7 per 100,000.

• Gonorrhea prevalence rates for women in 1989 was 234.1 per 100,000 population. The rate for black women was 1,411.2 per 100,000 and for white women it was 54.3 per 100,000.

Another bacterial infection that has outnumbered gonorrhea is chlamydia trachomatis. Owing to the lack of a national surveillance reporting system, the incidence of chlamydia is not known. However, data from physicians and surveillance projects estimate 34 million cases each year (Horton, 1992, p. 30). One complication associated with chlamydia infections is pelvic inflammatory disease (PID), which affects the fallopian tubes, causing scarring, which predisposes women to ectopic pregnancy. An African-American woman who has had several bouts of different or the same STDs, where treatment may have been delayed due to inability to pay, may be at serious risk for scarring of the fallopian tubes and ectopic pregnancy. Further reported by Horton (1992, p. 15), throughout the 1970s and 1980s, African-American women had more ectopic pregnancy maternal deaths than white women, and there were no reported deaths from ectopic pregnancies in 1987 in blacks. However, in 1989 the death rate from ectopic pregnancy among African-Americans was five times higher than among white women (Horton, 1995, p. 17). It was reported (*Challenger*, 1996) that actor/dancer Ben Vereen's sister died on March 14, 1996 from complications of ectopic pregnancy.

Continuous infections from other venereal diseases like genital herpes simplex infection (accounting for 30 million cases), genital warts (12 million cases), and HIV (1 million cases) all severely impact on the health status of African-American females. Infectious diseases are particularly threatening to the health status of African-American women, accounting for preventable illness (e.g., venereal diseases), changes in lifestyle behavior, and education. When combined with chronic diseases, health status is further compromised.

One lifestyle behavior is responsible for a variety of illnesses among African-American females. How severe is the problem? Braitwaite and Taylor (1992, p. 124) reported their findings regarding diabetes during a 1989 epidemiological research conference. They stated that black women had a higher prevalence of obesity, a strong factor for non-insulin-dependent diabetes mellitus (NIDDM). Among people with diagnosed diabetes, 82% of adults were black, obese women as compared with 62% of white women. Diabetes among African-Americans is almost two times higher than in white women, and in 1990 the age-adjusted death rate from diabetes in blacks was 25.4%, in white women the rate was 9.5% per 100,000 (Horton, 1995, p. 74).

Cardiovascular disease is two to four times more likely in women with diabetes. Heart disease is one of the leading causes of death among women age 55 and older, and for African American women, they are 55% more likely to die from heart disease than white women (Washington, 1994, p. 32). According to the Public Health Service report (1994), the death rate per 100,000 in 1989–1991 is higher for African-American women in all age groups. Contributing to the heart rate mortality is hypertension, which

Table 2
**Percentage of Women in the United States
with Hypertension by Race and Age, 1990**

Age	African American	White
18–29	4	4
30–44	15	7
45–64	41	23
65+	47	39

Source: *Women's Health Data Book* (Horton, 1995),
adapted from Figure 3-2, p. 58.

is twice as common in African-American women as in white women. In 1990 the percentage of women with hypertension increased in every age group (see Table 2).

For the African-American female, risk factors such as smoking, lack of exercise, high-salt diets, heavy fat intake, and stress must be controlled. Some doctors believe that there may be a link between heart disease and gynecological problems. African-American women have more external fibroid tumors and undergo more hysterectomies, both of which can cause damage to the estrogen-producing ovaries. According to Edward Copper, MD, president of the American Heart Association, "this can result in a big drop in estrogen, leaving the heart more vulnerable" (Washington, 1994).

Because African-American women tend to delay seeking care, they are often poor surgical risks. Furthermore, there is some evidence that medical treatment may be curtailed owing to inability to pay for invasive life-saving procedures (e.g., bypass surgery). As you can see from Table 3, in 1988 cancer was the second leading cause of death in African-American women.

For most of the leading causes of death, African-American women have the highest death rate, as seen in Table 4.

Although the rate for cancer has been better for women than men between 1980 and 1989, the age-adjusted death rate for breast cancer increased by 12% for African-American women, while it remained steady for white women. As a consequence, in 1989 cancer mortality was 14% higher for African-American women than for whites—26.0 and 22.9 death rate per 100,000, respectively (Reed et al., 1993, p. 36). And for other cancer sites,

mortality from stomach cancer is 1.5 times greater . . . than white . . . ; and they are three times as likely to have cancer of the esophagus and 2.5 times as

Table 3
Leading Causes of Death in African-American and White Women, 1988

Cause	African-American	White American
Heart Disease	1	1
Cancer	2	2
Stroke	3	3
Pneumonia/Influenza	6	4
Chronic Obstructive Pulmonary Disease	11	5
Accidents	5	6
Diabetes	4	7
Suicide	20	12
HIV/AIDS	14	24

Source: Women's Health Data Book (Horton, 1995), adapted from Table 3-3, p. 45.

Table 4
Age-Adjusted Cause of Death, Rate per 100,000 Population for African-American and White Women

Cause of Death	African-American	White
Heart Disease	165.5	100.7
Cancer	136.3	111.2
Stroke	41.0	22.8
Pneumonia/Influenza	13.5	10.2
COPD	11.3	16.1
Unintentional Injuries	19.9	7.0
Diabetes	25.7	9.6
Suicide	1.9	4.8
HIV/AIDS	12.0	1.3

Source: Women's Health Data Book (Horton, 1995), adapted from Table 3-1, p. 54.

likely to die from the disease than white women. . . . Both mortality and incidence rates for cervical cancer are 2.5 times higher among black females than white females: Black females have 33% excess death rate from cancer of the corpus uteri as compared to white females (p. 37).

Between 1980 and 1992 the age-adjusted death rate increased 16% for black women while it decreased 5% for white women; the age-adjusted death rate for breast cancer for black women was 24% higher than the rate for white women. (USDH&HS, 1994, p. 3). Equally, the age-adjusted lung cancer death rate for women continued to increase for both black women and white women between 1980 and 1992 (p. 3).

Lupus, a disease of the immune system, affects women nine times more than men and is three times more prevalent among African-American women than white women (*Women's Health Data Book*, Horton, 1992, p. 58). Lupus is a chronic illness that is difficult to diagnose. Systemic lupus erythematosus (SLE) is the most severe form of the disease. An illness like SLE may require multiple clinic visits that, for millions of uninsured African-American women, could mean late diagnosis and delay in treatment, resulting in poor outcomes.

Alcohol use among African-American women is another serious problem. In one study cited in the *Women's Health Data Book* (Horton, 1992, p. 78) it stated "that despite the overall lower reports of use, black alcoholic women who were followed for 12 years after treatment were found to have higher mortality rates than white alcoholic women in the same study" (6.7% versus 3.9%). African-American women also report more alcohol-related health problems than white women, such as cirrhosis, esophageal cancer, and hepatitis. Furthermore, fetal alcohol syndrome among African-American infants is reported to be disproportionately higher when compared to other ethnic groups, ranging from 0.3 per 10,000 births for Asians, 0.8 for Hispanics, 0.9 for whites, and 6.0 for blacks, with Native Americans having the highest rate at 29.9 as reported in a study by the National Institute on Drug Abuse (Horton, 1995, p. 106). Illicit drug use among African-American women is also an abuse (NIDA, 1990) as presented below:

• Almost 8 million (36%) blacks have used marijuana, cocaine, or other illicit drugs at least once in their lifetime.
• Black women are more likely than women of any other racial/ethnic group to use crack.

African-American women are disproportionately affected by the AIDS virus, primarily through their illicit drug use. As Horton (1992, p. 38) reports, these women experience major exposures to AIDS through injectable drugs (55%), followed by heterosexual contact (34%). Of the AIDS deaths in 1990, 46% of the women who died had been exposed to injectable drugs (p. 36). By 1994 the rate of infection was 16 times higher among African-American women than white women (POZ, 1995, p. 78). It has been estimated that there will be between 165,000 and 215,000 persons who will die from AIDS in the next several years. A vast number of them will be African-American women.

Some estimate that in America, on any given day, there are 4.6 million persons who are suffering from some form of mental disorder like depression (discussed in more detail later). Mental disorders are often related to substance abuse (17%), anxiety (15%), and depression (8%) (Horton, 1995, p. 82). One illness that seems to be pervasive in African-American females is depression. There are approximately 7 million women in the United States with diagnosable major depression (Horton, 1995, p. 82), whose cause can be due to biological factors (e.g., menstrual cycle, menopause) or psychosocial factors (e.g., limited social roles and racism). Depression among African-American women was the subject of a six-month study at five sites—Baltimore, New Haven, St. Louis, Piedmont, Calif., and Los Angeles. For obvious reasons (O. J. Simpson and Rodney King) I have selected the results of the Los Angeles site for review. Major depression among black and white women is not uncommon. In the 25–44 age group, depression in blacks was 14% and in whites, 6% (Horton, 1995, Table 4-3, p. 87). Lifetime prevalence of major depression among black and white women (1980–1983) in the 25–44 age group is of concern. The percent of cases of depression for blacks was 30% and for whites, 14% (Horton, 1995, Table 4-4). Life crisis, unemployment, sexism, poverty, high-stress jobs, single parenthood, coupled with overt racial discrimination, all make African-American women particularly vulnerable to depression. One result of severe depression is suicide. Of the 31,000 suicides in 1991, white men committed the majority of the reported cases. For African-American and white women, the age-adjusted suicide rates in 1991 were 4.8 and 1.9, respectively. Also, in 1991, among African-Americans aged 15–24 and 25–44, suicide ranked seventh and tenth, respectively (Horton, pp. 89–90).

In this commentary I have presented some of the acute, chronic, and common health practices that impact on the health status of African-American women. Also presented are some of the social factors (e.g., poverty and racism) that also affect African-American women. Some of the social indicators that impact on the health of these women will be presented in more detail in the chapters that follow. Excessive deaths in the African-American community are attributable to many factors. However, poverty and access to health services and health care providers must be considered as some of the opposing variables to optimal health status. Obviously we cannot deal with every variable that impacts on the health and social status of African-American females. However, attention has been drawn to those variables that need to be looked at with a questioning eye.

WORKS CITED

Beardsley, E. (1990). Race as a factor in Health. In Rima Apple, ed., *Women, Health and Medicine in America: A Historical Handbook*. New York: Garland.

Centers for Disease Control (CDC). (1992). *HIV/AIDS Surveillance Report*. Atlanta: CDC.

The Challenger (1996). Death of Ben Vereen's sister probed. March 27, p. 4.

Harper, A. & Lambert, L. (1994). *The Health of Populations: An Introduction*, 2nd ed. New York: Springer.

Hoffman, F. L. (1897). *Race, Traits and Tendencies of the American Negro*. New York: Macmillan.

Horton, A. J., ed. (1992 and 1995). *The Women's Health Data Book: A Profile of Women's Health in the United States*. Washington, DC: The Jacobs Institute of Women's Health.

Leffal, L. D. (1990). "Health status of black Americans." In *The State of Black America*. New York: National Urban League.

National Institute on Drug Abuse (NIDA). February, 1990.

POZ STATS (1995). New York: POZ Publishing, August/September.

Reed, W., Darity, W.; & Roberson, N. (1993). *Health and Medical Care of African Americans*. Westport, CT.: Auburn House.

U.S. Department of Health and Human Services, National Center for Health Statistics (1994). *Health U.S. 1993: Public Health Services*. Hyattsville, MD.

U.S. Bureau of the Census (1992). The black population in the United States, March 1991. *Current Population Reports*, Series P20-N464. Washington, DC: U.S. Government Printing Office.

Washington, H. A. (1994). Heart & Soul Informer, *Heart & Soul*, Spring, 32–34.

Wegman, E. M. (1990). Annual summary of vital statistics 1989, *Pediatrics*, 8,(6), table 4, p. 841.

Wegman, E. M. (1993). Annual summary of vital statistics 1992, *Pediatrics*, 92,(6), table 4, p. 747.

PART I

HEALTH ISSUES

1

Allowing Illness in Order to Heal: Sojourning African-American Women and the AIDS Pandemic

Reneé Bowman Daniel

The AIDS pandemic presents one of the most unique medical and social dilemmas of our time. This is especially true for African-American women who are suffering from the silence of AIDS and dying in the shadows. Imagine, HIV/AIDS is the leading cause of death for African-American women of childbearing age in New York and New Jersey, and, we comprise 72% of the women's population diagnosed with HIV/AIDS. How reflective of the cultural and historical struggle that has enslaved a community for centuries, as we have allowed ourselves to be postured as pillars of strength, healers, and caretakers for everyone but ourselves. As a result of adopting an edifice of strength based on the denial of our own illness, we now suffer the consequences that endanger the very goal we sought to achieve: the continuation of the people.

This chapter will examine, from an Afrocentric perspective, the sociocultural factors that surround the pandemic of HIV/AIDS among African-American women. The chapter presents the concept of empowerment for wellness for the collective survival of African-American women and the community in which they are a centerpiece. Recommendations and strategies are profiled that will "allow illness in order to heal."

HIV/AIDS is killing us. Our community, our women, our men, our children, our families, our futures are besieged by a tragedy happening in silence. HIV/AIDS, cast as the health catastrophe of our lifetime, and originally characterized as an epidemic of gender (male) and sexual orientation (homosexual), is disproportionately claiming the future of African-Americans. Demographically, African-Americans make up 12.3 percent of the U.S. population yet are disproportionately represented among the poor, the homeless, and those with indicators of poor health status. Our median age is 27.5, the median household income is $18,098, and nearly one-third of African-Americans live below the poverty threshold (Hale, 1992). So is this pandemic of HIV/AIDS but just another expense of life in America?

JUST THE HIV/AIDS FACTS

Although the overall number of AIDS cases reported in 1994 (80,691) declined from the number reported in 1993 (106,618), the Centers for Disease Control and Prevention reports 58,428 cases of acquired immunodeficiency syndrome among adult and adolescent women (13 years and older). The proportion of cases among women has steadily increased from 7% in 1985 to 18% in 1994. Acquired immunodeficiency syndrome and other illnesses due to HIV infection have been the fourth leading cause of death among women in the United States ages 25–44 since 1992 (CDC, 1994). Among AHANA (an acronym for African-American, Hispanic, Asian American, and Native American), African-American lives are claimed at a rate six times higher than any other group.

Carrying the burden of the increase are African-American women and children. According to Land (1994, p. 356), "urban mortality rates indicate that acquired immunodeficiency syndrome is the leading cause of death among African-American women between the ages of 15 and 44 years of age." The 1994 AIDS case rate per 100,000 population for adult and adolescent women was 62.7 for African-Americans in comparison with 3.8 for Caucasians. African-American women's HIV infection cases totaled 10,218 in 1994 in comparison to 4,075 for Caucasian women. African-American women acquire AIDS at a rate of 14 times higher than Caucasian women. Information from the HIV Survey in Childbearing Women found that an estimated 7,000 HIV-infected women gave birth to infants in 1993. Assuming a perinatal HIV transmission rate of 15–30%, this translates to 1,000–2,000 infected infants born during 1993 alone (CDC, 1995).

Currently in New York State acquired immunodeficiency syndrome is the leading cause of death among African-American children ages one to four. Compounding this is a mean survival rate for African-Americans once diagnosed with AIDS of 8 months compared to 18 to 24 months for Caucasians. As Richie (1994, p. 184) states, "statistics indicate that the most frequent mode of transmission of the HIV virus to African-American women is through sexual contact with African-American men who were intravenous drug users and or gay, or bisexual." Heterosexual contact with an infected partner or a man at high risk for HIV infection accounts for 38% of AIDS cases in U.S. women and it is expected to become the primary means of spreading HIV infection in most industrialized countries over the next several decades. By the year 2000, the number of worldwide AIDS cases of women will begin to equal men (CDC, 1995).

Since 1981, when the first case of a woman with AIDS was reported in the United States, very little attention has been paid in clinical practice, research, or public discussion to women and the HIV/AIDS epidemic. The first National Conference on Women and HIV infection, held in December 1990 and sponsored by the U.S. Public Health Service (PHS), found that little was known about women and acquired immunodeficiency syndrome. What we do know is that the overall health status of African-Americans is alarming. The National Center for Health Statistics reports that African-Americans are far more likely to be assessed in fair or poor health than any other racial group, and the rate of disease among African-Americans is almost double the rate of other races. African-Americans are generally 1.5 times as likely to be sick and die as Caucasians (Avery, 1992; U.S. DHHS, 1985).

In the last three years of the 1980s, public health officials reported increases among African-Americans in diseases that had been steadily declining since the beginning of the century, and considered on the verge of eradication less than a decade ago. Many of these diseases are virtually unknown in middle-class or wealthy neighborhoods. They include tuberculosis, hepatitis A, measles, mumps, whooping cough complicated by ear infections, and, acquired immunodeficiency syndrome. The leading causes of death among African-American women are heart disease, cancer, stroke, chronic obstructive pulmonary disease, pneumonia, diabetes, chronic liver disease, and, acquired immunodeficiency syndrome (CDC, 1990).

So what's wrong with this picture? This is the twentieth century, yet the health status among African-Americans and particularly African-American women reflects the historical and environmental structures of the pre–Civil War era. (Lawson & Thompson, 1994). It has been 132 years since the Emancipation Proclamation, yet African-American women are still held in bondage. For so long our strength, love, and determination have been focused on the welfare of our community. We have been taught to reorder our own priorities and to find enrichment through our commitment to the welfare of others. We are the wives, partners, daughters, sisters, and mothers of a community plagued by illness and the pandemic of acquired immunodeficiency syndrome, but we ourselves are also losing in the AIDS battle (Sharp, 1993).

To understand the phenomena of African-American women suffering and dying in the shadows of a worldwide pandemic, our community must begin to understand the plight of the African-American women's cultural and historical legacy, the disempowering concept of illness as it is perceived in our community and family structures, and remember the successes of our struggles in this land we call our home. It is only then that we will be empowered to act expeditiously to heal and embrace a healthy community.

LIVING AND DYING IN THE SHADOWS

African-American women share a cultural and historical legacy that not only provides African heritage, but also encompasses a life of exploitation and oppression through colonization, enslavement, codified apartheid, de facto segregation, or other expressions of individual and institutional racism. In a world that is dominated by "isms" such as racism and sexism, the African-American female suffers from her status of being black and female. This is further compounded if she is a single parent in a society where the two-parent family is perceived to be the "norm."

To be part of the African-American, black, Afro-American, negro or colored community means a yoking to racist stereotypes that associate our community with criminal or deviant behavior. Much of the salient social science literature, written by others about our African-American community, proliferates the European American myth about our lack of morality and our hypersexuality. Utilizing race as the relevant label of identification, black people are seen in a positive domain only in terms of good athletes, musicians, dancers, rhythm and blues and jazz singers, jokesters, and unskilled laborers—in other words, servants to the majority culture. And what of the African-American female's image of herself and her life?

A survey conducted by the National Health and Nutrition Examination Surveys (NHANES) found that over half of the African-American women participants between the ages of 18 and 25 report living in a state of psychological distress (Avery, 1992).

Historically, sexism has played a major role in robbing us of our self-esteem and devaluing our femaleness. Pre–Civil War bondage found African-American women treated as organic property, denied the right to their virginity, and cast in the role of breeder and sex object, ready for use at anyone's leisure. Post–Civil War bondage placed African-American women in a unique juxtaposition of prostitution and prostration. Medical care was provided because we were economic assets. However, the medical care and practices were predicated on physiological differences rooted in a racist ideology that believed in the genetic inferiority of black women.

Today, African-American women continue to find definition in the context of human relationships through which we take on the role of nurturer, shoulder the burden of caretaker/giver, and affix ourselves as helpmate. We are celebrated for our unique devotion to the task of mothering, our innate ability to bear tremendous burdens, and for our ever increasing availability as sex objects (hooks, 1981). Now let us add to this the myth of the black matriarch. This theory casts African-American women as both dominating and castrating, idealizes the strength, liberation, assertiveness, and self-sufficiency of the matriarch, who is responsible for the survival of the family and the community, while, within the same breath, blaming the black matriarch for the so-called disintegration of the African-American family (Staples, 1994).

Make no mistake, this divisive theory espoused by social scientists really only serves to emasculate our men and our community, and to provide the impetus for the African-American women's sojourn into a life of self-denial and self-blame. Seen as this monument of strength, the African-American woman is left with little room to be ill or have any problems, engage in help-seeking behaviors, or utilize resources.

We do not allow ourselves to be ill. Many have recognized the cultural and societal dynamics in the African-American community that allow us to distance ourselves from illness and this pandemic of acquired immuno-deficiency syndrome, which in many ways is like every other health, social, and economic crisis that African-Americans have faced for generations. Our impulse to distance ourselves from HIV/AIDS is less a response to AIDS than a reaction to the myriad of social issues that surround the disease and give it meaning (Dalton, 1989). African-Americans have been and continue to be blamed for the origin and spread of the acquired immuno-deficiency syndrome. After all, hasn't it been theorized that HIV/AIDS originated in Africa, and because of their sexual prowess Africans contributed significantly to the spread of the virus/disease?

Compound a deep-seated suspicion and mistrust for a health system that recognizes African-Americans as subjects of programs to reduce fertility and demonstrate the effects of untreated disease and I would say the denial and rejection of the illness is a buffer between a hostile environment and the community.

Illness is not a welcomed concept in the African-American community. One speaks more of being "sick," for this is tolerated although not acceptable. Illness is an experience, a complex set of ways in which the sick person, the members of the family, and other social networks understand, live with, and respond to the symptoms and disability (Kleinman, 1988).

Being ill is disruptive because it impinges on our sense of who we are and our important social relationships. HIV/AIDS, although fitting the definition of a disease, "a biophysical condition," is also an illness. As an illness it is often experienced as overwhelming, unpredictable, and uncontrollable because it paralyzes the person's ability to manage life, to plan, and to act.

The human response to illness is to give it meaning, to interpret it, to reorder upon socially available categories from a large cultural repertoire and from personal and family stories and meanings absorbed from our particular ethnic and religious backgrounds. In the case of minor illnesses, the interpretations might include our underlying definitions of health and illness, and our notions about why we get sick and how to get well. Seriously disruptive illnesses are likely to evoke further interpretations about the meaning of life, moral responsibility, suffering, relationships, and death (Freund & McGuire, 1991, p. 157).

Acquired immunodeficiency syndrome in the general population has been interpreted as the "gay" disease, followed by the conclusion that this is "God's way of ridding the earth of undesirables," under which category the community places intravenous drug users. Under what category should we place the African-American woman, and/or her child?

How does the community come to understand that she is now sick, dying because she perhaps loved another, whose history or present lifestyle includes drug abuse, needle sharing, or a bisexual/homosexual relationship? Can we be strong enough to allow an illness that is robbing the community of it's childbearing force?

Can we admit that the African-American woman who has been the centerpiece in the struggle for equality, dignity, and honor and has contributed to every scene of the African-American drama (Ashante & Mattison, 1991) might have to step down from her role as caregiver and become a vessel needing care. And are we as a community ready to truly understand the relationship between love and sexuality and African-American women's role, position, and status in intimate relationships? This understanding is necessary to begin to undo the "blackface" of acquired immunodeficiency syndrome.

Sexual relationships between men and women have often been identified by the female gender in terms of obligations: it was the woman's duty. However, the social dynamics of the African-American woman's sexual experience placed her in the position of being seen as excessively sexual and promiscuous. As the mainstream culture promoted repressive attitudes toward sexuality, rooted in group value systems and practices manipulated by racism and sexism, the African-American community banished the extremely subjective and stigmatized experience of sexuality to a position of silence. Therefore, African-American women do not have experience with acknowledging or sharing with one another or their mates the interconnections of our emotional, sexual, and reproductive experiences. In essence, we have become disempowered through our own historical and contemporary experiences, and we cannot allow or acknowledge illness, particularly those emanating from our sexual experiences.

ALLOWING ILLNESS IN ORDER TO HEAL

Our community is under attack by what has been identified as the health catastrophe of our lifetime: acquired immunodeficiency syndrome. It has a divide-and-conquer strategy that is not new to the African-American community. However, as we continue to struggle for life, progress is often threatened by a weakening of our social and personal resolve (Billingsley, 1992). Despite these situations and daily experiences that continue to oppress our community, we continue to be an unconquered people whose strength is found in our interdependence, our collectiveness, and our sense of peoplehood. We must remember, though, to be unconquered is not synonymous with faring well. As Dalton (1989, p. 219) points out, "we have been so busy expressing our fears that we have failed to express our hopes." We must draw strength and advantage from the situations that oppress us because that is how we have made substantial gains and progress in our community in the past.

The concept of empowerment for well-being must be reenergized in the African-American community. The African-American woman must redefine her status and reclaim the importance of self. She must remember that it is through her visions and dreams that our people have been kept alive. Now in the midst of this pandemic, the African-American woman finds herself once again "the centerpiece in the struggle for equality, dignity and honor," and her survival and the survival of our people will require a refocus, a readjustment, and creative health promotions and life-saving program initiatives.

But how do African-American women in particular begin the process of empowerment that must be thoroughly integrated into everyday life experiences and situations? How do feelings of powerlessness translate into action or inaction on African-American women's health issues? How does a person, long denied the right, begin to believe she has a right to allow illness in order to heal (Avery, 1992)?

REFOCUS, READJUSTMENT, AND ATTITUDINAL CHANGE

Treatment of all women relative to HIV/AIDS will be more effective if it is based on an understanding of the societal context in which women live as well as women's relational needs. The community must perceive and understand the consequences of a disempowered state with which an African-American woman quietly lives, as well as other life issues that contribute to her inability to protect herself from infection. These include psychosocial, cultural, and legal barriers to her decision making; the lack of economic alternatives, with the consequent dependence on a man for support; the societal role of women as primary caretakers of children, husbands, and parents; the well-known case of women's lower literacy in some countries, their limited mobility, and limited access to information; and let us not forget societal attitudes about sexuality (Williams, 1991). Health promotion and prevention efforts have to a great extent centered on educating women about "safe sex," but advising women to use condoms truly reflects a lack of knowledge about gender role and power issues within the African-American community.

African-American women must be able to see themselves in any proposed preventive service models, and to see myself I must understand how this program will benefit my children, my companion(s), my community. African-American women are more likely to become sensitized to AIDS issues, to engage in empowering behavior such as HIV testing, to encourage prophylactic use, and to have an enhanced perception of HIV risk if the messages stress culturally relevant values. Such values include linking behavior change to pride in one's culture, noting the adverse effect of acquired immunodeficiency syndrome in African-American communities, and stressing family responsibility to protect the children (Land, 1994; Kalichman et al., 1992). Prevention efforts should focus on those methods that women can control: the use of spermicides and physical barrier methods of protection that also serve as contraception, such as diaphragms and cervical caps. Additionally, service providers must refocus prevention efforts on educating our men and include grassroots community involvement that will encourage men to talk with one another about their sexual behavior (Avery, 1992). When we can stop punishing our women, our men, and our children for their behavior and provide life-saving information in an atmosphere of trust, perhaps the community attitude about HIV/AIDS will change.

Our community is long overdue for an attitude adjustment that will serve as the precursor to behavioral change. We must change our attitudes about ourselves. No longer do we have the time or the circumstances in which we can allow others to usurp, manipulate, exalt, degrade, alter, exploit, suppress, or turn back against African-American women, our image of self and of our community. Avery (1992, p. 37) also argues that "we must stop loving our sons and raising our daughters and give both the love needed for responsible self respect."

Perhaps then African-American women and men will develop the atmosphere in which conversations can occur regarding those issues that impact upon the health of the community, such as a roof over our heads, a meal on the table, dignity and self-worth, quality health care, the education of our children, economic stability, self-determination, and sexual intimacies and behaviors and their consequences.

We must understand that the stereotypes about our moral character and hypersexuality are convenient racist and sexist labels that lead to a socialization process that pits us against our men and holds the community hostage by way of mental enslavement to the concept of deviance and the recurrent fear of further stigmatization.

The African-American community must learn that labels dictate process, and that to empower our community to accept an illness in order to heal we must engage in a dissociative relationship with current labels and classifications. Our messages, our literature, the physical environments of our programs, and our communities must focus on old terms that have more acceptable meanings and circumstances. Instead of using the words "sick" or "ill," we need to promote the concept of "healthy" and "unhealthy" communities, families, men, women, and children. This concept is without stigma yet personal enough so one can link health to the welfare of the community. We must organize around the promotion of a healthy community focusing on those facts and actions that inform and educate rather than blame and victimize. In the African-American community we believe in "calling a spade a spade," so tell it like it is in a language without labels.

The African-American community is unhealthy at present because there is a condition one can acquire that will stop the body's immune system from protecting it from all the different viruses, infections, and diseases that are in our environment. The future of our community is being jeopardized by a condition called acquired immunodeficiency syndrome. The use of this language first teaches by actually describing the condition. The use of the actual medical term promotes the demystification, lessens the stigmatization, and removes the label of deviance from this "illness." The African-American community accepts conditions, as typified by the terms high blood pressure versus hypertension, sugar versus diabetes. It is all a matter of words and their symbolism.

TEACHING A COMMUNITY OLD TRICKS

There has always been and continues to be tremendous strength in the African-American community. Perhaps it is time to ask ourselves: how have we survived? As directions and paths are forged at this most significant crossroads, let us not forget to investigate and then celebrate the remarkable successes that so many women and families have experienced, and learn from these in order to progress in the face of ever more pressing obstacles. To build a healthy community, service providers, whether indigenous or professional, must utilize a holistic approach—a comprehensive family systems treatment approach that views the family as a whole, focuses on relationship building, and demonstrates care for African-American women in all their roles. Our African-American community must implement and then evaluate community interventions that will prevent further transmission of acquired immunodeficiency syndrome and target women who are at high risk.

Educational outreach and condom distribution, as well as teaching drug addicts how to clean their needles, or offering a free "needle exchange" program have proved effective in reducing the rate of HIV transmission. This type of intervention has proved effective in Zaire, where prostitutes were given condoms and free treatment for sexually transmitted diseases and their annual incidence of HIV infection decreased from 18% to 3% in just over two years (Garcia, 1993). The National Black Women's Health

Project (NBWHP), established in 1990, is another example of innovative programming efforts. Additional creative partnerships must be established with those organizations and institutions that have a natural place in the community.

The single most influential resource in the U.S. African-American community is the black church. It is imperative that the church become more involved in outreach and intervention efforts, recognizing that true empowerment comes through teaching of the holy scriptures as given to us in the *New World Translation of the Bible* (1984, p. 1416), Romans 10: verses 14 and 15:

However, how will they call on him in whom they have not put faith? How, in turn, will they put faith in him of whom they have not heard? How, in turn, will they hear without someone to preach? How in turn will they preach unless they have been sent forth?

The Health Resources and Services Administration (HRSA), Bureau of Health Resources Development (BHRD), sponsored a two-day Work Group on Barriers to HIV Care for African-Americans living with HIV disease. Nineteen African-American participants and six federal representatives discussed issues related to the barriers in providing HIV/AIDS services to African-Americans and possible strategies to reduce or eliminate these barriers. Several of the participants in the work group were people living with HIV disease.

When developing programs, the consumers of the service are an integral part of the design process. Within the African-American community, positivism is crucial. Subsequently, the name of the program should be positive and support self-empowerment rather than identify the problem. Program materials should be multicultural and give evidence of an understanding of the different cultural interpretations of common expressions. They should also be Afrocentric by design and reflect our own standard of beauty and color. HIV/AIDS is killing us. Are we to succumb? A nation is not conquered until the hearts of its women are on the ground. Then it is done, no matter how brave its warriors or how strong its weapons. We have the right and, above all, we have the duty to bring strength and support of our entire community to defend the lives and property of each individual family (Robeson, 1958). Despite murders, rapes, and suicides, we survived the middle passage, and the auction block did not erase us. Not humiliation, nor lynchings, nor individual cruelties, nor collective oppression were able to eradicate us from earth (Angelou, 1986). What about HIV/AIDS? Will it get the hold on us? Of the seven areas for proposed technical assistance and evaluation studies identified by the HRSA Work Group (1994), the following three provide charge to the call:

1. *Identify characteristics of information systems that work for African-*

American communities. Persons desiring to have an impact on the current status of health in our community must recognize the tradition of oralism in the African-American community and use this tradition/custom as a component in any intervention strategy. One must understand the implications of the relationship between human and spiritual support systems in the African-American community and employ an information system that utilizes these networks.

2. *Identify resources of and for African-Americans and develop a directory of services and skills and a dissemination plan.* The concept of equifinality as a systemic process of change is one that must be taught and understood by service providers and the consumers of their service. What are the answers to how are we currently dealing with this AIDS pandemic in our communities? What programs, services, grassroots efforts, and individual efforts are having a successful impact, and can they be modeled?

3. *Identify characteristics of effective organizations.* Often we are so busy working in the "trenches" we do not look up to see how we are staving off the war, to determine and evaluate why what we are doing is successful, and to re-create the success. We do know that effective service providers operate under a system of inclusion.

WORKS CITED OR USED

Angelou, M. (1986). *All God's Children Need Traveling Shoes.* New York: Random House.

Ashante, M. K. & Mattison, M. (1991). *Historical and Cultural Atlas of African-Americans.* New York: Macmillan.

Avery, B. Y. (1992). The health status of black women. In R. Braithwaite and S. E. Taylor, eds., *Health Issues in the Black Community.* San Francisco: Jossey-Bass, 35–51.

Billingsley, A. (1992).*Climbing Jacob's Ladder: The Enduring Legacy of African-American Families.* New York: Simon & Schuster.

Centers for Disease Control. (1990). *Cases Selected Notifiable Disease.* Morbidity & Mortality Weekly Report. Washington, DC: Department of Health and Human Services, 39, 704–707.

Centers for Disease Control (1994). *HIV/AIDS Surveillance Report, Year End 1994.* Rockville, MD.

Centers for Disease Control (1995). *Recent Trends in Reported U.S. AIDS Cases.* Rockville, MD, March.

Dalton, H. L. (1989). Aids in blackface. *Daedalus,* 118, 205–227.

Freund, P. & McGuire, M. (1991). *Health Issues and the Social Body: Critical Sociology.* Englewood Cliffs, NJ: Prentice Hall.

Garcia, A. (1993). HIV positive, church negative. *Diatribe,* Spring (People of Color News Collective) Berkeley, CA.

Hale, C. B. (1992). A demographic profile of African Americans. In R. Braithwaite & S. E. Taylor, eds., *Health Issues in the Black Community.* San Francisco: Jossey-Bass, 6–19.

Health Resources and Services Administration. (June 1994). Work Group on HIV/ AIDS Health Care Access Issues for African Americans. Rockville, MD.

hooks, bell. (1981). *Ain't I a Woman: Black Women and Feminism*. Boston: South End Press.

Kalichman, S., Hunter, T., & Kelly, J. (1992). Perceptions of AIDS susceptability among minority and nonminority women at risk for HIV infection. *Journal of Counseling and Clinical Psychology*, 60, 725–732.

Kleinman, A. (1988). *The Illness Narrative: Suffering, Healing and the Human Condition*. New York: Basic Books.

Land, H. (1994). Aids and women of color. *Families in Society: The Journal of Contemporary Human Services*, 6, 355–361.

Lawson, E. J. & Thompson, A. (1994). The health status of black women. In R. Staples, ed., *The Black Family: Essays and Studies*. Belmont, CA: Wadsworth.

New World Translation of the Holy Bible. (1984). Watch Tower and Tract Society of New York, Inc.

Richie, B. (1994). AIDS: In living color. In E. White, ed., *Black Women's Health Book: Speaking for Ourselves*. Seattle: Seal Press, 182–187.

Robeson, Paul. *Here I stand* (1958). In D. Winbush Riley, ed., *My Soul Looks Back, 'Less I Forget': A Collection of Quotations by People of Color*. New York: HarperCollins, 1991.

Sharp, Saundra. (1993). *Black Women for Beginners*. New York: Writers Readers Publishing.

Smith, L. & Thrasher, S. (1993). A practice for working with overwhelmed African American families. *Black Caucus: Journal of the National Association of Black Social Workers*, 25th Anniversary Issue, Spring, 1–7.

Staples, Robert. (1994). Social inequality and black sexual pathology. (1994). In R. Staples, ed., *The Black Family*. Belmont, CA: Wadsworth, 341–349.

U.S. Department of Health & Human Services. (1985). *Report of the Secretary's Task Force on Black and Minority Health*. Washington, DC: U.S. Government Printing Office.

Williams, P. (1991). A new focus on AIDS in women. *ASM News*, 57(3), 133–134.

2

Lupus: The Silent Killer

E. Ginger Sullivan

Nelson Mandela (1994, p. 751) was speaking about more than political freedom when he recently wrote: "Freedom is indivisible; the chains on any one of my people were the chains on all of them, the chains on all of my people were the chains on me." Disease can, and does, limit our freedom by enslaving all people. Regardless of our place or position in the world, whether as physician, nurse, medical student, advocate, or patient, one way to maximize freedom is to fight the chains placed upon us by disease and disability. We can remove those chains by fighting disease as an informed health professional, a united family, and as a concerned community. In this chapter I will urge that health professionals understand the warning signs of lupus, employ a full range of medical and social treatments upon diagnosis, address lupus as part of a larger battle against minority health disparities, and advocate more research for minority and women's health issues, particularly for additional biomedical research efforts on lupus.

LUPUS AS A WOMEN'S HEALTH ISSUE

Women's health issues are tragically understudied. As a result, huge disparities in health status exist, with women suffering higher incidences of some diseases than men, especially African-American women, with little known about how and why these disparities take place. One such example is systemic lupus erythematosus (SLE), a multisystem disorder of the immune system, involving an attack on the body's natural tissue. More than 500,000 people in the United States have lupus, and perhaps that figure is closer to 1 million. Hundreds of thousands of people suffer from lupus worldwide. The annual incidence of patients with SLE in the United States is 7.6 cases per 100,000. The prevalence rate in the United States is one in 2,000. However, the incidence of SLB is extremely disproportionate: in the United States, 1 in 700 for women between the ages of 20 and 64, and 1 in 245 for African-American women of the same age group.

Virtually every physician will encounter at least one case of SLE at some point while in practice. Little is known about the origin or causation. Genetic factors are strongly suggested. Hormonal factors are also suspected, since women have a higher incidence of the disease and approximately 30% of females with lupus undergo exacerbation of symptoms during pregnancy or the postpartum period. Environmental factors may also be important: SLE may flare up after viral infection, ultraviolet light exposure, surgery, stress, or ingestion of some foods. Treatment is important, effecting a decline in morbidity and mortality. Currently, more than 90% of lupus patients in the United States now survive at least 15 years. However, there is a widespread ignorance about lupus, especially in our community. Even its name reflects that ignorance. In Latin, *lupus* means wolf and *erythematosus* means redness. The name was first given to the disease because it was thought that the skin damage resembled the bite of a wolf.

THE NATURE OF LUPUS

Lupus is a stealth disease—a disease often missed because of its deceptive, complex nature. Its cause is unknown; the results devastating, if untreated. Lupus should be easily diagnosed because it is characterized by the presence of a variety of autoantibodies. However, it is often misdiagnosed because of the diversity of its clinical manifestations, including oral ulcers, arthritis, serositis, renal disorder, neurological problems, and other disorders.

Lupus is a type of blood disorder, a disease in which the immune system of the patient becomes overactive, producing an excess of blood proteins (antibodies). These antibodies, in turn, attack healthy tissues in the body, inducing inflammation, redness, pain, and swelling in the affected parts of the body. As a result, the patient's joints, skin, kidneys, lungs, heart, or brain may be damaged. The symptoms of lupus differ from one person to another, making the disease hard to diagnose. Lupus is often mistakenly missed, as other causes are examined. Because of this, lupus is often called the "great imitator." According to the National Institute of Arthritis and

Musculoskeletal and Skin Disease at the National Institutes of Health, the common signs of lupus are:

- red rash or color change on the face, often in the shape of a butterfly across the bridge of the nose and cheeks;
- painful or swollen joints;
- unexplained fever;
- chest pain with breathing;
- unusual loss of hair;
- pale or purple fingers or toes from cold or stress;
- sensitivity to the sun; and/or
- low blood count.

Other signs of lupus can include mouth sores, unexplained convulsions, hallucinations or depression, repeated miscarriages, and unexplained kidney problems.

The cause of lupus is unknown. Biomedical researchers have not yet isolated the specific sequence of events that trigger the overactivity of the immune system. In fact, our understanding of lupus is evolving, with sometimes conflicting results (Mills, 1994). But we do know that in some people lupus becomes active after exposure to sunlight, infections, or certain medications.

Also, lupus is not catching. A patient cannot transmit it to someone else. It is not a form of AIDS or cancer. However, lupus has a tendency to show up within families, where more than one person can have lupus. It should be considered a risk factor for families where lupus has previously appeared.

Lupus affects mainly young women, often between the ages of 15 and 44. It is also disproportionately found in African-American women at a rate three times higher than white women. As many as one in almost every 250 African-American women will have this disease.

A CASE STUDY

It is important to listen to those with lupus. Each story is different, and each person's needs must be recognized and addressed. It is a fundamental mistake to treat people with lupus as if they are patients processed through medical offices or clinics on a conveyor belt. Lupus patients—indeed, all patients—need the full and specialized attention of each health professional they encounter.

In preparation for this chapter, I listened to a friend of mine who confronts lupus, an attractive African-American woman who has lived with this disease for over 30 years. She is decidedly upbeat about those three decades, because she has fought and won a battle against disease fatigue, depression, and cultural ignorance.

I asked her to describe the physical symptoms of lupus. She stressed to me that each patient manifests different symptoms. In her case, she experienced chronic fatigue, chills and fever, joint pains accompanied by swelling, a skin rash on her face and elsewhere on her body, edema, upper respiratory and other bacterial/fungal infections, and many additional problems that affected her kidneys, lungs, spleen, central nervous and endocrine systems. She also found the emotional trauma to be quite severe, with long periods of depression due to the manifestation of the disease, the extensive use of medication, strained relationships with family members and friends, battles with health insurers to maintain coverage, negotiating with the bureaucracy administering Social Security disability payments, struggles to continue employment, and long periods of hospitalization. Medication use was also linked to hair loss and weight fluctuations.

In an attempt to regain some control over her life, my friend found that she had to make certain decisions to provide the maximum amount of freedom possible in her circumstances. She discovered that a prerequisite to maintaining some level of independence was choosing a medical practitioner who was competent, sensitive with patients, and understanding. She found that word of mouth was often the best source of information about the performance of physicians and other health professionals. She found that a good dermatologist was important. She also recommended finding competent hair care specialists.

My friend wisely stressed that lupus patients need to establish an exercise schedule, in order to build up and maintain strength. Of course, such a schedule may not be possible for some patients, and may have to be abandoned during periods of difficulty by almost all patients. But any exercise is better than none, and the payoff is during times of enforced bed rest and when medication begins to adversely affect the body.

Mental health is an important consideration. So she urges all lupus patients to develop a hobby to fill the days and to occupy the mind. There will be long periods of hospitalization. Good mental health depends on diverting the mind from enforced idleness or destructive forms of self-reflection.

There are also many challenges on the job. Patients must realistically determine their ability to function with even a reduced workload. Decisions must be made about with whom to confide. Even if they don't know, concerned office workers will ask questions. Employers will also ask questions, and a person with lupus must decide how much to tell an employer, perhaps running the risk of losing the job because of potential medical costs and reduced job performance. My friend felt that the best approach was to become even more attentive to appearance and work performance, demonstrating that a person with lupus can effectively continue her employment. However, she also felt that the employee should reduce her workload, and that personal guilt about not finishing work should be diminished.

Above all, patients must strive to be hopeful. My friend has found that hope is the best medicine. Many people find hope through religious beliefs; others find it through a philosophy of life. Others find it through the love and joy of family, friends, and neighbors. I was struck by one statement made by my friend: "I believe the Creator provides each of us the support we need. I'm glad mine was through my family. I can't imagine living with lupus without them."

People are living with lupus. All of us must help them to cope. Mental health experts should urge that denial be overcome. But that doesn't mean patients should resign themselves to the disease. They must fight back with all the physical, social, religious, emotional, and cultural tools at their disposal. For those of us without lupus, we have the potential to become part of the support that enables people to live with the disease. We can join in the daily fight of thousands of people who are living with lupus this very day.

DIAGNOSIS

Symptoms are varied, and no two people have the same symptoms. So diagnosis is often difficult, and usually must be made over an extended period of time. The skin rash is usually an important symptom. If there is any question, a skin biopsy can help in the diagnosis. A sample of skin tissue may reveal deposits of antibodies and complement proteins. A kidney biopsy also may show deposits of antibodies and immune complexities. The Lupus Foundation of America has also argued that the following tests can aid in diagnosis:

- The antinuclear antibody test can determine if the patient has antibodies that react with components in cell nuclei. Over 90% of lupus patients will have a positive reaction to the test. Unfortunately, positive tests also occur with a variety of other diseases and in up to 10% of the normal population.
- The anti-DNA antibody test determines if the patient has anti-bodies to DNA.
- The anti-Sm antibody test looks for antibodies to a protein that was first discovered in the blood of a lupus patient. While many lupus patients do not have anti-Sm antibodies, they are rarely found in people without lupus.
- Tests for the presence of immune complexities (the combination of antibodies and the substances with which they react) in the blood are valuable both for diagnosing and monitoring the disease.

• An analysis should be made of the serum complement level, which tends to fall when the disease is active. The serum complement level is a group of proteins involved in the inflammation that can occur in immune reactions.

The interpretation of these results can be problematic due to the unpredictable nature of the disease. For instance, a test can be positive one time and negative the next, depending on whether the disease is active or in remission (Stehlin, 1991).

TREATMENT

Treatment for lupus is usually determined by the individual manifestations of the disease. However, no treatment cures the disease. Depending on the particular difficulties encountered by each patient, treatment through pharmacological intervention can help to address the symptoms and can lead to remission. For example, arthritis and serositis are often controlled by aspirin or other nonsteroidal antiinflammatory drugs. Many of the dermatological manifestations are addressed by use of hydroxychloroquine and quinacrine, except for panniculitis and skin problems caused by arteritis. Patients should use sunscreen and avoid intense exposure to the sun.

A moderate dose of glucocorticoid is often used to counter thrombocytopenia and hemolytic anemia. When thrombocytopenia is resistant to glucocorticoid therapy, then danazol, intravenous low dose vincristine, cyclophosphamide, or splenectomy are used. However, because of the risk of infection, a decision to undertake a splenectomy should be weighed very carefully (Mills, 1994).

I must stress that lupus is a complex disease, with singular manifestations. Each patient must be treated for the specific symptoms. There is no standardized formula or one-size-fits-all solution (Mills, 1994).

MEDICAL EDUCATION'S CONTRIBUTION

Dr. Donald Girard (1994, p. 6), commenting on medical training for internal medicine, recently suggested broad changes in the residency program curriculum. These changes would be most appropriate for assisting medical students to understand, recognize, and treat lupus. Dr. Girard believes that "traditional training in internal medicine has failed to provide either the curriculum or the atmosphere that allow for appropriate teaching of issues unique to women's health." Solutions, which should generally be adopted throughout the many disciplines of medical training, would include better clinical curricula and continuing medical education, improved methods to teach sensitive approaches to African-American women's health, and efforts to break down perceptions of persisting discrimination against women in the medical professions. In addition, students should familiarize themselves with the many resources now available on lupus. Some of these resources are listed at the end of this chapter.

USER-FRIENDLY HEALTH SYSTEM

In order to effectively employ early diagnosis and treatment of African-American women with lupus, health professionals must work to make the health care system more "user-friendly." The human dimension in health care must not be forgotten. If programs are provided, we should work to make them available to those who qualify. Important services cannot only be available during the normal business day. When confronted with a choice between staying at work or seeing a physician, many people stay on the job. A more practical arrangement can be offered, such as earlier or later clinic operating hours, or weekend openings.

Health professionals must also treat with dignity those who seek medical assistance and recognize culturally sensitive issues related to the African-American female. They cannot be indifferent, rude, unconcerned, or hostile because they failed to recognize those who are distrusting of their care. African-American women who come into the system are often confused, frightened, despairing, and in need of a friend. White physicians who will treat the majority of African-American women with lupus need to greet them with understanding, compassion, and respect. If this kind of treatment is not provided, the patients will be discouraged and driven away—disenfranchising them as surely as if the doors were locked.

Therefore, outreach and community involvement become crucial, perhaps central, parts of the health care system. Health care professionals must also work "beyond the four walls" of the hospital, clinic, or office. Many years ago, hospitals provided most of the medically intrusive services needed by patients. But now, with the advent of outpatient services and with the use of new medical technologies, the health care system has evolved into a more diversified, more dynamic, and more competitive environment. As a result, health professionals must become more aggressive and visionary in providing less costly, quality health care to those in need. Health professionals must interact more closely with patients through communitywide nutrition programs, through outreach services to African-American communities, through placement of clinics in housing projects and other underserved areas, through special efforts to address HIV infection and tuberculosis, through health partnerships with businesses and schools, through health fairs and career counseling, through mobile services in vans and trailers, through help-lines and radio programs, and through establishment of patient information services with telecommunications networks.

MORE RESEARCH AND INFORMATION CAMPAIGNS
ARE NEEDED

More research is essential to understand the cause or causes of lupus. As well, public information campaigns are essential, but at the moment are practically nonexistent. Research and information campaigns should be expanded as part of a comprehensive effort, thereby addressing disparities in the health status of African-American women and between the general population. Such efforts should be immediately initiated in the United States. By taking these steps, we can increase the health status of African-American women in general and enhance longevity of thousands of African-American women who are not yet diagnosed with lupus.

There is a vital need for additional efforts to address reproductive health problems, breast cancer, osteoporosis, and other difficulties disproportionately, or exclusively, encountered by African-American women. I was pleased that during my husband's (Louis W. Sullivan, MD) tenure from 1989 to 1993 as U.S. Secretary of Health and Human Services, he worked with the Congress in 1990 to establish an Office of Research on Women's Health at the National Institutes of Health (Pinn, 1992). This was a hopeful and necessary first step toward focusing more resources on women's health needs. But much more remains to be done.

For instance, women need to craft and disseminate a loosely unified vision of the equality of men and women. In many countries, including the United States, women are still regarded as second-class wage-earners, prohibited by glass ceilings and office politics from making greater strides in the workplace. But this vision of equality must also reflect at least one inequality: that men and women, while deserving the same respect, do not have the same health needs. In fact, our bodies are not the same—a fact that is still not fully recognized by the health care system, even though a freshman course in biology would clearly make a prima facie case for difference. True equality and respect for all people must include a greater proportion of resources devoted to women's health, a point often made in national and international forums, such as the International Conference on Population and Development in Cairo, the World Summit on Social Development in Copenhagen, and the United Nation's Fourth World Conference on Women in Beijing. The August 1995 issue of *Science* was devoted to women's health research, indicating that the women's health movement is an emerging American and global political force, propelled by exclusion from clinical trials, ignorance of a female perspective in the design of these trials, and the paucity of important areas of biomedical research on women's health, such as cardiovascular disease, AIDS, and depression (Hurtley & Benditt, 1995). An additional, and central, problem is that the health of women in the Third World is seriously at risk, especially from complications due to childbirth, cardiovascular disease, and AIDS. In a *JAMA* editorial, Vivian Pinn (1992, p. 739) offers the view that equity in biomedical research is good science, good medicine, essential fairness, and morally correct. She observed:

The challenge now inherent in women's health research is to establish a scientific knowledge base that will permit diagnosis and effective prevention and treatment strategies for all women, including those of diverse cultural and ethnic origins, geographic locations, and economic status. The ultimate objective is good science to enhance biological wisdom and inform the development of policies and medical standards from which women and men can benefit equally.

Establishing equality in biomedical research will require a "paradigm change," a change of linking and a change of priorities (Sechzer et al., 1994). But such a change is long overdue and essential if the health care system is to successfully diagnose and treat lupus.

In this chapter, I have argued for greater awareness of lupus, which will lead to earlier diagnosis and treatment. By offering a full range of medical and social interventions, lupus patients can often lead comparatively normal, productive, and full lives. With a growing recognition of lupus and its pervasive effect on African-American women, the health care system must address health disparities in our African-American communities and between genders, both in the United States and around the world. Health care is a common concern for all people, and good health is one road to freedom and equality.

Yet, while it is imperative that we fight lupus, this is just one of many diseases that demand our attention. The long road to good health and freedom is a difficult journey. But we cannot fail to stay the course. When the complexity and enormity of our work together becomes burdensome, perhaps we can find inspiration from a former political prisoner, who describes the arduous travel ahead:

I have walked that long road to freedom. I have tried not to falter; I have made many missteps along the way. But I have discovered the secret that after climbing a great hill, one only finds that there are many more hills to climb. I have taken a moment here to rest, to steal a view of the glorious vista that surrounds me, to look back on the distance I have come. But I can rest only for a moment, for with freedom come responsibilities, and I dare not linger, for my long walk is not yet ended (Mandela, 1994, p. 751).

APPENDIX: ADDITIONAL RESOURCES

For further information, patients and health professionals may wish to contact one or more of the following organizations:

The American Lupus Society
260 Maple Court, Suite 123
Ventura, CA 93003
800-339-0443; 800-331-1802; 805-339-0467 (fax)

Lupus Foundation of America, Inc.
4 Research Place, Suite 800
Rockville, MD 20850-3226
301-670-9292; 800-558-0121

Lupus Foundation of Greater Washington
515 A. East Braddock Road, Suite 2C
Alexandria, VA 22314
703-684-2925

I also recommend the following pamphlets/papers for patients:

Edmund DuBois and Mavis Bowen Cox, eds., "Lupus Erythematosus: What Is Lupus? What Causes Lupus? Symptoms and Course of Lupus, Diagnosis of Lupus, Incidence Lupus," American Lupus Society, Ventura, CA 93003.

Leslie Epstein and Bonnie Romoff, "So Now You Have Lupus: An Aid to Understanding the Psychological Aspects of Lupus," available from the American Lupua Society, Ventura, CA 93003.

Graham R. V. Hughes, "Lupus: A Guide for Patients," American Lupus Society, Ventura, CA 93003.

NIAMS Task Force, "What Black Women Should Know About Lupus," National Institute of Arthritis and Musculoskeletal and Skin Diseases, National Institutes of Health, Box AMS, 9000 Rockville Pike, Bethesda, MD 20892.

Daniel Wallace, Bevra Hahn, and Francisco Quismorio, "A Patient's Guide to Lupus Erythematosus," American Lupus Society, Ventura, CA 93003.

WORKS CITED

Girard, E. D. (1994). Women's health care: Is American medicine failing on many fronts? *The Internist,* February, 8–10.

Hurtley, S. & Benditt, J. (1995). Women's health research: A special report. *Science,* 269, 729–892.

Mandela, N. (1994). *The Long Walk to Freedom.* London: Little, Brown, 1994.

Mills, A. J. (1994) . Systemic lupus erythematosus. *The New England Journal of Medicine,* 300 (26), 1871–1879.

Pinn, V. (1992). Women's health research: Prescribing change and addressing the issues. *Journal of The American Medical Association (JAMA),* 268, 14.

Sechzer, A. J., Griffin, A. & Pfafflin, S. (1994). Women's health and paradigm change. In *Forging A Women's Health Research Agenda: Policy Issues for the 1990s, Annals* of the New York Academy of Science, 736.

Stehlin, D. (1991). Living with lupus. DHHS Pub. No. (FDA) 90-3178. A reprint from *FRD Consumer* magazine, December 1989–January 1990. U.S. Department of Health and Human Services, Food and Drug Administration. Washington, DC: U.S. Government Printing Office.

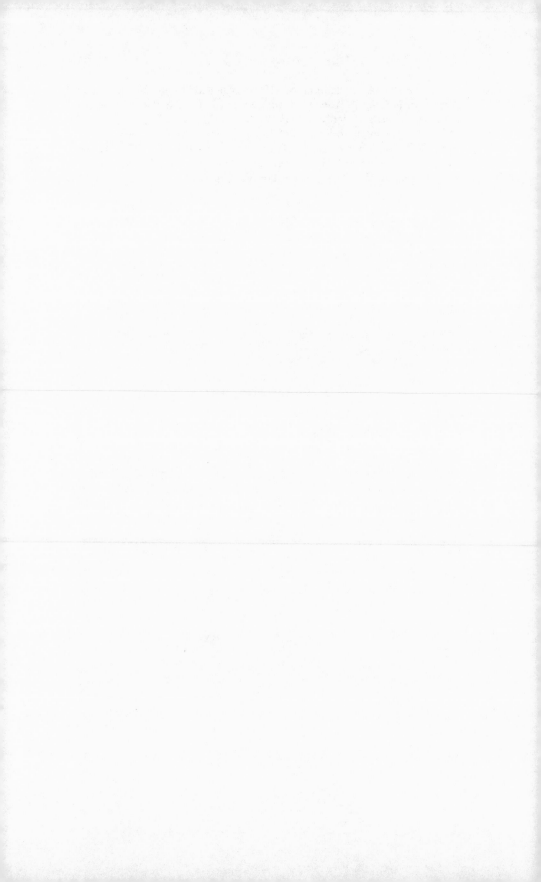

3

Exploring Health Issues and Health Status of African-American Women with Emphasis on Cancer

Noma L. Roberson

For the past decade, the African-American female population has captured the attention of researchers, social scientists, health practitioners, and public health professionals who have sought to understand their cultural uniqueness in respect to health care. The needs of African-American women have generated serious concerns and stimulated research on women's issues. Unfortunately, the majority of studies about African-American women have failed to thoroughly investigate various cancer-related issues for this population segment. Rather, studies have focused on issues related to acculturation into the dominant society. Equally important, only a few studies have attempted to explore health issues and health status of African-American women with respect to cancer.

It is the devastating impact of cancer on the African-American female population that warrants attention in this area. In particular, the increase in mortality rates and the poor survival rates have emerged as critical over the past several years. Because the risk of cancer may be strongly associated with lifestyle and behavior, cultural values, and belief systems, researchers have sought to conduct preliminary studies about the causal and/ or contributing factors.

While there may be a number of critical issues about African-American women's plight with health and illness that need attention, three major issues were selected for discussion in this chapter: (1) African American women's placement in the social structure that influences health and illness; (2) societal stereotypes about African-American women's health-related behavior; and (3) the health status situation of African-American women that impacts disease occurrence.

Research about African-American women's health must be grounded in their views, definitions, and concerns lest health care research continues to render inaccurate and biased views based on inappropriate categories generated secondhand by persons not a part of those worlds (Olesen, 1977).

The purpose of this chapter is to discuss issues and health status as each influences the occurrence of cancer among African-American women. This chapter will consist of four sections, three of which will focus on selected issues about health care and cancer among African-American women. The fourth section will include implications and future recommendations for research.

In this chapter, the term "African-American" will be used to mean persons whose lineage includes ancestors who originated from Africa (Water, 1991). The term "black American" has been used in the United States to distinguish these persons from those of European origin without such ancestry. It is important to note this trend because national data for cancer statistics refer to black Americans rather than African-Americans. Thus, the terms African-American and black Americans may be used interchangeably throughout the discussion.

AFRICAN-AMERICAN WOMEN'S PLACEMENT IN THE SOCIAL STRUCTURE

To know African-American women's placement in the social structure is to understand who these women are and their family roles, the effects of ethnicity on sociomedical attitudes and behaviors, and the social patterning of health and illness. These are factors that help to influence women's decision-making and attitudes necessary to become participants in primary and secondary health care.

African-American women are unique persons known for their strength, support, and survival skills. While they are similar in this respect, African-American women are not a homogeneous group. There are variations in educational levels, religion, and socioeconomic status, region by region and group by group. African-American women are represented in every socioeconomic group in the country. Unfortunately, a large portion of African-American women live at or below the poverty level. Many live in central cities, in areas typified by poverty, poor schools, crowded housing, unemployment, violence, and high levels of stress. Constant plights with these situations result in suffering and a change from balanced health to illness. The effects that African American women suffer are nowhere more telling and more significant than in mortality rates and life expectancy (Reed, Darity, Roberson, 1993). Mortality rates and life expectancy among African-American women will be discussed later in the chapter.

To further enhance the reader's understanding about African-American women's placement in the social structure, it is important to examine the African-American family. It must be stated that family stability is a trademark of West African societies, where most of the forebears of America's black population originated. The primary family model of Western Africa was the consanguineal model. Like those in other parts of the world, African families embody two contrasting bases for membership: consanguinity, which refers to kinship that is commonly assumed to be biologically based and rooted in blood ties, and affinity, which refers to kinship created by law and rooted in "in law" (Suderkasa, 1981).

The African family system was characterized by "respect, restraint, responsibility, and reciprocity." The family structure was built on a mutual respect of women, men, and children. The uniqueness of this system can be seen in the way family relations and women are handled (Smith, 1985). "Excepting those areas where Islamic traditions overshadowed indigenous African traditions, women had a good deal of control over the fruits of their own labor" (Suderkasa, 1981). Wives exhibited more power and influence than did their European sisters.

Whatever the relative strengths or weaknesses of the West African family structure, it must be remembered that people of African heritage were also forced to face the holocaust of slavery. Slavery systematically attempted to destroy the African-American family (Smith, 1985). Over several hundred years, every attempt was made to strip them of home, dignity, and culture.

African-American women's morals were greatly affected as they were systematically raped by white slave masters and forced to bear unwanted children (Smith 1985; USDHHS, 1990). In a search for the cause of many types of cancers believed to be related to lifestyle and behaviors, there has been a failure by researchers to take a serious look at the impact of slavery demands on African-American women's attitudes, beliefs, and health practices. These are, no doubt, key factors to the introduction of cancers of the female reproductive organs. A description of contributing risk factors supports this thesis (American Cancer Society, 1995; USDHHS, 1985).

Slavery enforced the equality of black men and women through equal pain. The slave master did not treat slave women with any of the respect and daintiness with which he treated white women. Slave women were forced to work in the fields alongside of men. They were punished with equal severity and the physical realities of pregnancy and pre- or postnatal care were never considered as reasons for time out from work.

When the West African concept of respect for women is coupled with the way women were forced into positions of equal suffering during slavery, the matriarchal argument takes on a new light. The severe economic pressures of post-Reconstruction America forced African-Americans to adopt whatever ways were necessary to survive. "Adapt" was what African-Americans did to survive slavery (Smith, 1985). It was also the way that African Americans handled their plight. As demeaning as it was, African American women took whatever work was available in order to survive and prevent racism from destroying the family totally. This speaks to the issue of female-centered households, which does not necessarily suggest male weakness. Rather, it suggests that in the face of extraordinary pressure, the African-American family has somehow found the strength to survive (Smith 1985; Dodsom, 1981).

The family system is the apparent foundation for social patterning. For the sake of discussion, much can be said about social patterning. It appears that social patterning was parallel to the developing family unit and crisis situations that primarily stemmed from slavery. As slavery shaped African Americans' plight into class distinctions and racial differentiation, it resulted in their social, economic, and political disadvantage.

A question that warrants discussion is whether peoples' placement in social structure is linked to their health. Perhaps the relationship between social structure and health may be seen by considering the physiological effects of the social environment. The social environment—people and their interactions with each other—affects physiological and health processes (Insel & Moos, 1994; Levine & Scotch, 1970). Holmes and Rohe (1967) found that events leading to significant change can lower an individual's resistance to disease. They studied several populations and found a significant relationship between the extent of life changes and the time of disease onset. The striking consistency in the distribution of mortality and morbidity between social groups may explain this phenomenon. For example, the more advantaged groups—whether expressed in terms of income, education, social class, or ethnicity—tend to exhibit better health than other members of their societies. This distribution is not believed to be bipolar (i.e., advantage versus disadvantage), but, rather, graded so that each change in the level of advantage or disadvantage is, in general, associated with a change in health.

This social patterning of health is important for a number of reasons. First, the graded relationship between health and social position may suggest hypotheses concerning the etiology of both specific disease and all-cause mortality. Second, the size of the gap between mortality rates of the advantaged and disadvantaged groups gives some indication of the potential for improvement in a nation's health. Third, identification of the groups who are at greatest risk of poor health can inform sound governance of medical services. Fourth, understanding the causes of social variations in health should lead to intervention strategies that can reduce them (Blone, 1995).

Another area of discussion in respect to African-American women's placement in social structure, the effect of ethnicity on sociomedical attitudes and behaviors, is well-known and has been documented for many years (Berkanovic & Reeder, 1973; Suchman 1964). Researchers believe that ethnicity can serve as a useful moderator variable in identifying relatively homogeneous subgroups of individuals with similar cultural beliefs and values. Ethnic groups have been shown to differ in utilization patterns, concepts of illness and disease, and interaction with mainstream health professionals and organizations (Harwood, 1981). Although ethnicity may be relevant to health beliefs and behavior, the relative effect of ethnicity on preventive health behavior must be separated from the simultaneous effect of socioeconomic status. Ethnic groups that are characterized by low income, limited education, and ethnic segregation oftentimes have a decreased awareness of preventive health measures and less access to medical care (Schreiber & Homiak, 1981).

According to Reed et al. (1993), health and illness are distributed across populations in predictable ways. The relative proportions of good or poor health among individuals may be directly related to those individuals' placement in the social structure. Of all the inequalities in the distribution of health, one of the most pronounced is the distribution by race.

Over the past decade, the target audience for many health and medical care programs has been racial/ethnic groups (e.g., African-Americans, Hispanics, and Native Americans). Limited knowledge about many aspects of health and illness among various racial/ethnic groups, along with limited skills for planning and implementing health services, are reasons for limited success to impact disease rates.

Mistakenly, African-Americans have generally been labeled as low-income and "hard to reach"—a perjorative term often applied to audience segments based on their socioeconomic status, their ethnicity, or their level of literacy. Freimuth and Mettger (1990) critically examined the hard-to-reach label and looked at stereotypes associated with this label.

Low-income and hard-to-reach individuals often are depicted as both financially and psychologically impoverished, focused on short-term rewards, and, therefore, uninterested in pursuing preventive health behaviors and medical care. These individuals are labeled as less responsive to suggested health behavior changes because they are said to care less about themselves than persons of higher socioeconomic status and have minimal health knowledge to build on. Also, low-income individuals may be labeled as hard to reach because they have not adopted behavior change strategies at the rate of their middle- and upper-class counterparts.

In addition to dealing with the labels of low income and hard to reach,

African American women have also had to deal with the term "ethnic groups." According to Henderson and Primeaux (1981), this term refers to individuals who share a unique cultural and social heritage passed from one generation to another. It must be pointed out that ethnicity is not synonymous with race. Rather, race refers to a system of classifying humans into subgroups based on specific physical and structural characteristics (Freimuth & Mettger, 1990).

The hard-to-reach label is most frequently applied to African-American and Hispanic ethnic groups. This is most likely because these are the largest ethnic minority groups (USDHHS, 1985). This label is also likely to be applied because their cultures are different from and not understood by many who plan health care programs and conduct research for these groups. Finally, the hard-to-reach label was applied because of evidence from several health companies that African-Americans have low levels of knowledge about health issues, less positive attitudes, and make fewer behavioral changes than other audiences (Freimuth & Mettger, 1990).

In respect to low-literate populations as being labeled hard to reach, they are labeled as such because these persons cannot read printed material, the most widely available form of health information. Some authors contend that people with limited reading skills have underdeveloped information processing resources and are therefore confused by complex written and verbal medical instructions (Freimuth & Mettger, 1990).

Societal stereotypes about African-American women's health-related behavior observations over the past two decades showed that numerous stereotypes are associated with the hard-to-reach label. According to a report, the stereotypes can perpetuate myths about groups that may be discriminatory, fallacious, and patronizing. There are four common stereotypes used to characterize hard-to-reach audiences: fatalism, poor information processing skills, limited communication channels, and distrust of dominant institutions (Childers & Post, 1975).

Fatalism is a prominent stereotype applied to those labeled hard to reach. According to these authors, this stereotype suggests that a pervasive sense of helplessness impacts negatively on health status. The American Cancer Society's report, *Cancer and the Poor: A Report to the Nation* (1989), illustrated the relationships between fatalism and health status. The report quotes: "Based both on limited knowledge and the reality of their encounters with health care systems, poor Americans mistakenly believe that there is no hope of surviving cancer. Fear and misconceptions about cancer prevent many poor Americans from seeking needed care."

A second stereotype—poor information-processing skills—suggests that hard-to-reach audiences have low-level reading skills and may not possess basic communication skills needed for everyday transactions (Childers & Post, 1975). In addition, the audience may lack well-developed cognitive skills and problem-solving orientations. There is a further claim that those who are uneducated are uninformed, unexposed to new information, and tend to have difficulty learning when exposed (Feldman, 1966). Schatzman and Strauss (1955) assert that persons with poor communication skills tend to think in concrete rather than abstract terms and that their knowledge may be based on immediate experience.

Not only is there the belief that hard-to-reach audiences have underdeveloped information-processing skills, but that their information channels are restricted (Freimuth, 1995). According to this stereotype, a majority of the hard-to-reach groups reported frequent use of television and minimal use of print media (Freimuth, 1995). Thus, there tends to be an overreliance on electronic media and underexposure to health-related information that is largely available through print media. Further, the nature of the communication network of the hard-to-reach group is another part of the limited communication channels (Freimuth, 1995). Contact from the outside usually is limited. As a consequence, much misinformation is prevalent.

Distrust of dominant institutions is the fourth stereotype. This distrust is toward federal, state, and local government agencies. Lack of knowledge and utilization of services within these audiences stems not from a lack of information, but from a mistrust and even a deliberate rejection of the "establishment" position (McKnight, 1985).

While these four stereotypes characterize those who are hard to reach in terms of weaknesses, there are four alternative conceptualizations that emphasize strengths (Freimuth, 1995). First, there are the emphases of differences rather than deficits. The "difference thesis" argues that people from different social strata have the same underlying competence as those in the mainstream of the dominant culture (Mechanic, 1989). Further, it suggests that when individuals are motivated to acquire information and that information is functional in their lives, they will make use of it. By contrast, the deficit thesis assumed that the relationship between socioeconomic status (SES) and intellectual performance was caused by a deficiency of basic cognitive ability.

The second alternative conceptualization was "blame society rather than individuals" (Mechanic, 1989). Blaming the social system places the responsibility for change on the entire social system. Societal blame is the tendency to hold a social system responsible for the problems of individual members of the system. For example, the societal-system-blame perspective may focus on the tobacco companies for people's smoking habits, while the individual-blame perspective holds the individual responsible for his or her smoking behavior. Health promotional campaigns focus on the individual's dietary choices rather than going after the food manufacturers. Further, society emphasizes individual responsibility, assuming it is their duty to make appropriate lifestyle changes to reduce his or her risk of preventable disease.

The third alternative conceptualization for the hard to reach is "other advantage" (Lyons, 1972). Lyons suggests that to communicate successfully with hard-to-reach groups means to drop a characteristic, patriarchal stance and treat other cultures with dignity and respect. The term "other-advantaged" was suggested as a replacement for "disadvantage." Other-advantaged conveys a message that each individual experiences advantages and disadvantages in different aspects of his or her life.

The fourth alternative conceptualization involves a change in the notion of information and communication (Dervin, 1989). Instead of the traditional information-as-description model, Dervin offers an alternative conceptualization—that is, information-as-construction. She suggests that the information-as-description model implies that communication is a linear process. A source has the responsibility to transmit that information to people who need it. Communication must be conceptualized as all involved in creating meaning by establishing a dialog. The new approach advocated by Dervin was communication-as-dialogue. This approach suggests ways to understand how the audience members make sense of their everyday lives, and how their behaviors are linked both to messages they attend to and social structures they live in.

These four alternative conceptualizations appear to be the similarity in the emphasis on the importance of respecting the unique strengths that any audience brings to the health communication process, involving the audience in the communication process, and redefining communication as an active exchange between participants. Obviously there is no place for the hard-to-reach label for African-American women or any other minority group. The consideration of adopting alternative conceptualizations may result in more effective health care delivery to individuals regardless of race/ethnic identity.

HEALTH STATUS

Health and illness are distributed across all population groups in the United States. A pattern of health and illness can be found among racial/ethnic groups whereby some appear to fare better than others. Some groups have historical problems that have perhaps placed them at a disadvantage in terms of increased threats of illness and shortened life span. This appears to be the situation with African-American women.

Health is a consequence of social, economic, and political factors. According to Reed et al. (1993) "good health is an asset in the economic sense as well as the general sense." Healthy people are better able to compete in life and to obtain more desirable jobs. On the other hand, persons in poor health are less able to compete and often acquire less desirable jobs. The strong association between health and economic well-being suggests that people's status more or less predicts their health. A brief history of the status of African-Americans may shed light on health consequences and thus enhance one's understanding about the emphasis on cancer.

History about the status of African-Americans reported in a formal study dates back to 1944 when the Myrdal study, *An American Dilemma* was released (Myrdal, 1944). Gunnar Myrdal was recruited from Sweden to head this investigation. This work reigned for nearly a quarter of a century as the authoritative study of African-American life in the United States and became a classic in social science. There was no other competing major study.

The Myrdal study concluded that the racial oppression of African-Americans was a result of an American conflict, an American dilemma: the discrepancy between an egalitarian ideology and racial discriminatory behavior. While Myrdal addressed the real issue—racial oppression—he presented it in combination with a very positive statement about America, about an American creed, thereby making his overall assessment of racial problems more palatable to the reading audience.

It should be pointed out that African-American critics argued that the Myrdal study paid too little attention to institutional racism, and that the elimination of racial discrimination and domination would require addressing social structural problems and institutional change. Further, it was argued that in studying social problems it was important to examine the relationship between social problems and social structure. This study failed to investigate this issue.

Commissioned as an update of the Myrdal study, in 1984 the National Research Council (NRC) (National Academy of Science, 1984) began a study to report on the status of African-Americans from 1940 to the present, and on their future status. The major criticism about this study was the limited involvement of African-American scholars in the concept, utilization, planning, and development of the study, and the inclusion of a number of scholars who ruled out both the historical oppression of African-Americans and contemporary discrimination against African-Americans as a major influence to current conditions.

Critics of the NRC's study were further concerned about the ramifications of a major study of African-Americans in the ideological climate of the 1980s. There has been a dismantling of the Great Society programs and a cease-fire in the war on poverty. There was a concern that the NRC's study would serve to validate the 1980s trends toward limiting the role of government in addressing the ills of society, particularly those concerning race.

As a result of concerns about the results of Myrdal's and the NRC's studies and no further major scientific investigations about the status of African-Americans, a third study was launched in 1987 with final reports published in 1993. Thus, *The Assessment of the Status of African Americans* was initiated at the William Monroe Trotter Institute at the University of Massachusetts in Boston (Reed et al., 1993). Thirty-five African-American scholars were organized into study groups to analyze the status of African-Americans in each of six topic areas: education; employment, income and occupations; political participation and the administration of justice; social and cultural change; health status and medical care; and the family. The study consisted of the widest possible discussion of the present condition of African-Americans and the social policy implications of that condition. This brief history about the status of African-Americans serves to enhance the readers' understanding about a number of contributing factors that may explain their health status.

There is a consensus among researchers that African-American women are at a disadvantage in terms of their health status (Institute of Medicine, 1985). This seriousness of health status is shown in national data through mortality rates and life expectancy (Reed et al., 1993; USDHHS, 1985; National Academy of Science, 1984). Overall assessments of the nature of types of disease patterns for cancer among African-American women are available. The difficulty lies in assessing health problems among this population group because of the failure to control the socioeconomic status and other quality-of-life indicators. The changing composition of the African-American family, the increasing number of female heads of households, the anticipated adverse effect on their health status, and changes in health care policies about special population groups make such data more vital than ever (USDHHS, 1985). A review of the sociodemographic characteristics including socioeconomic status of African-American women may help to explain some of the realities that influence their health status as well as other quality-of-life indicators.

African-Americans generally incur higher mortality rates than whites from all disease causes, including cancer, and show higher rates of other indicators of morbidity (American Cancer Society, 1995). Socioeconomic status is related to these differentials, as it has long been associated with health status for all races and with the health of African-Americans in particular.

Sorlie and colleagues (1995) presented an interesting scenario in respect to socioeconomic factors and health. These authors recognized that socioeconomic factors encapsulate complex information about a person's life. For example, several mechanisms could account for the relationship they found between length of education and adult mortality. The maternal and cultural resources of the parental home are strong predictors of a child's educational attainment. Therefore, education will be a marker of conditions during childhood, and these could determine adult health. Educational attainment is also a strong predictor of occupation and labor market position during adulthood, and these could be the major influence on adult health. The level of education might affect receptivity to health education messages, with adult health determined by the likelihood of adopting health-enhancing behaviors and quitting those that are health-damaging. Personality characteristics such as time preference or self-efficacy may independently influence both educational attainment and health behavior. Finally, poor health during childhood and adolescence could result in both low educational achievement and impaired adult health. In sum, many causal pathways are plausible and technical issues limit the infallibility (Sorlie et al., 1995).

African-Americans comprise the largest minority group in the United States. In the 1990 census, African-Americans numbered 30 million or 12% of the total U.S. population (U.S. Bureau of the Census 1992, 1993; O'Hara et al., 1991). African-Americans tend to be a younger population; reside primarily in the larger central cities of the South, Northeast, and Midwest; have less formal education; have lower individual and household incomes; and are more likely to be poor (USDHHS, 1985; USDHHS 1994a).

African-American women make up more than 50% of the adult African-American population. These women tend to have more children at earlier ages than white women. Nearly 50% of African-American women have incomes below the poverty level, compared with 25% of white women. Some 38% of African-American women are heads of households. These women are at a disadvantage because of the inability to find work and lower earnings (USDHHS, 1994b).

The most comprehensive indicator of patterns of health and disease, as well as living standards and societal development, is life expectancy of a population at various ages. Life expectancy is a hypothetical measure that indicates the chances of survival beyond certain ages if current age-specific mortality rates for an actual population were to continue. Therefore, it becomes a useful measure for comparing the mortality experiences of different populations (USDHHS, 1994a).

Records show that at the beginning of the 20th century, life expectancy at birth for African-Americans was 33.0 years (National Center for Health Statistics, 1992). By the middle of the 20th century, life expectancy had risen by 28 years to 60.7. Thereafter, life expectancy at birth increased more slowly, reached a peak of 69.5 years in 1984, and then declined to 68.8 years in 1989. In 1990 the life expectancy for African-Americans was 69.1 years. The life expectancy is 75 years for the general population.

In 1990 African-American life expectancy at birth was 9.1 years longer for females than for males (73.6 years versus 64.5 years) (National Center for Health Statistics, 1992). The survival advantage among African-American females born in 1990 continued a trend of increasing divergence in the life expectancies for African-American males and females. In contrast, whites have shown a steady decline since 1970 in the female survival advantage (American Cancer Society, 1995).

An African-American female aged 15 in 1990 could expect to live an additional 60.2 years, or 9 years longer than her male peer. A 45-year-old woman could expect to outlive a man of similar age by 6.2 years (32.4 years versus 26.2 years). Also, a 65-year-old woman could expect to outlive a man the same age by 17.2 years (17.2 years versus 13.2 years) (USDHHS, 1994a; National Center for Health Statistics, 1992). Some of the differentials in life expectancy among African American women and men may be explained by the high mortality risks for younger African American men.

The differential in life expectancy among selected age groups (e.g., 45 to 64 and 65 and older) can, in part, be explained by the experience with chronic diseases, cancer being one example. The specific role of the chronic diseases that exert a major impact on longevity and the quality of life among African-Americans may be examined from the perspective of mortality rates (National Center for Health Statistics, 1992).

Mortality data are used to identify the leading causes of death among subgroups (National Center for Health Statistics, 1992). By examining sex, age, and cause-specific mortality rates by race/ethnic groups for the most important chronic diseases, researchers and health care planners can determine how best to address the need to increase the span of healthy life for African-Americans and how to reduce health disparities among all Americans. The focus is on middle-aged and elderly populations because the burden of premature death from chronic diseases and the opportunities for prevention and control are greater among people in these populations than among persons in younger populations.

According to two national reports (USDHHS, 1994a; National Center for Health Statistics, 1992), the top three causes of death from chronic disease among African-American women aged 45 to 64 are ischemic heart disease (IHD), lung cancer, and breast cancer (142, 75.4, and 75 per 100,000 persons, respectively). IHD is also the leading cause of death among women 65 and older, followed by stroke and diabetes, and lung, colorectal, and breast cancers (1,085.8, 480.9, 227.5, 156.1, 142.6, and 130.4, respectively, per 150,000 persons) (USDHHS, 1994a). As indicated, three major cancer sites are among the leading deaths for African-American women.

The next section will focus specifically on cancer in African-American women, including disease prevalence by site and risk factors.

CANCER

Cancer is a disease that has a major impact on American society. It is the second leading overall cause of death in the United States, surpassed only by cardiovascular disease, and accounts for one out of every five deaths nationwide (American Cancer Society, 1995). Cancer is not one disease; rather, it is a constellation of more than 100 different diseases, each characterized by the uncontrolled growth and spread of abnormal cells (American Cancer Society, 1995; USDHHS, 1994a).

National data show that the incidence of cancer has been increasing throughout the population (Miller et al., 1993). Over the past four decades, however, cancer deaths increased at a much faster rate among the African-American population than among the Caucasian population (American Cancer Society, 1995; USDHHS, 1985; Miller et al., 1993; Boring et al., 1992). For example, during a 30-year period, the cancer death rate rose 10% for African-American women and virtually no change was seen in Caucasian women. Consequently a previously white predominance in cancer incidence and mortality prior to 1950 has been replaced by a black excess in incidence and mortality during the latter half of the century. In 1990 the incidence rates were 439 per 100,000 for African-Americans and 406 for Caucasians. The mortality rates were 228 for African-Americans and 170 for Caucasians (American Cancer Society, 1995). Cancer mortality is higher in African-Americans than in all races for several reasons, including higher rates of new disease (incidence), later stage at diagnosis, and poorer survival experience (Boring et al., 1992). Changes in disease statistics can be the result of a number of additional factors, including treatment advances, changes in disease detection, and the availability of technology. It is likely that a combination of these factors may explain what might represent a true increase in cancer incidence and mortality (American Cancer Society, 1995; Boring et al., 1992). Further, the difference in cancer death rates between African-Americans and Caucasians may be attributed, in part, to the relatively higher percentage of socioeconomically disadvantaged among African-Americans (Murphy et al., 1995).

The five-year survival rate for cancer in African-Americans diagnosed from 1983 through 1990 was about 40%, compared with 56% for Caucasians (American Cancer Society, 1995). A considerable part of this difference in survival can be attributed to late diagnosis. In 1995 a total of 120,000 cancer cases is expected to be diagnosed among African-Americans in the United States, many of whom will be African-American women (American Cancer Society, 1995).

Incidence and mortality statistics will be presented for African-American women to provide a measure of the burden of cancer in this population group. In descending order of incidence rates, the most common cancers among African-American women are breast, lung, colorectal, and uterine cervix. Some of these increased rates are believed to be related to socioeconomic differences reflected in lifestyle and behaviors that contributed to cancer risk, such as dietary patterns, tobacco and alcohol use, and sexual and reproductive behaviors. A discussion about four common cancer sites among African American women follows.

Breast Cancer

Cancer of the breast is the most common cancer among American women, including African-American women (American Cancer Society, 1995; Miller et al., 1993; Boring et al., 1992). The breast cancer incidence rate in American women increased from 85 per 100,000 persons in 1980 to 112.3 in 1987 (Murphy et al., 1995). Breast cancer incidence rates for American women have increased about 2% a year since 1980, but recently have leveled off at about 110 per 100,000 persons (Murphy et al., 1995).

National data show that overall incidence rates for African-American women was 17 percent lower than that for Caucasian women (93.1 versus 112.1 per 100,000 persons from 1986 to 1990) (Miller et al., 1993). This is shown in Table 5. The trend over the last few years appears to signal the expected turnaround in breast cancer incidence, based on the assumption that the increase during the 1980s was due, in part, to the increased use of mammography, allowing the detection of early-stage breast cancer before it would become clinically apparent (American Cancer Society, 1995).

Breast cancer mortality among African-American women continues to be higher than among Caucasian women, in spite of the fact that Caucasian women age 45 and older have higher incidence (Miller et al., 1993). For women under age 50, the breast cancer mortality rate decreased nearly 11% from 1973 to 1990 due to the decreasing trend in Caucasian women. In African-American women, under age 50, breast cancer mortality has increased by 2.5% over the same time period. Age-adjusted mortality rates for breast cancer were 30.8 per 100,000 persons for African-American

Table 5

Age-Adjusted Incidence and U.S. Mortality and Five-Year Survival Rates for Cancer by Site and Time Period for Black and White Women

Site	Incidence 1986–1990		Mortality 1986–1990		Five-year Survival 1983–1989	
	Black	White	Black	White	Black	White
Breast	93.1	112.1	30.8	27.3	64.1	80.5
Cervix	14.3	7.9	6.9	2.6	57.0	69.1
Lung & Bronchus	43.1	40.2	29.4	29.8	13.0	16.0
Colon & Rectum	46.8	40.9	20.6	16.0	48.9	58.7

Note: Incidence and mortality rates are for 100,000 population, are adjusted to the 1970 U.S. Standard Population Survival rates, and are expressed as percents.

Source: Miller et al. (1993).

women, compared with 27.3 for Caucasian women (Miller et al., 1993).

The five-year survival rate for localized breast cancer has risen from 78% in the 1940s to 93% today, if diagnosed at an early stage. If the cancer has spread regionally at the time of diagnosis, however, the five-year survival rate is 73%, and for persons with distant metastases the rate is 18% (American Cancer Society, 1995). Unlike the survival of many other cancers that may level off after five years, survival after a diagnosis of breast cancer continues to decline beyond the five years. The most current data show that 63% of the women diagnosed with breast cancer survive 10 years and 56% survive 15 years (American Cancer Society, 1995). Survival rates for African-American women continue to be poorer compared with Caucasian women, 64.1 versus 80.5 per 100,000 persons for the time period between 1986 to 1989 (Miller et al., 1993).

According to the American Cancer Society (1995), the risk of breast cancer increases with age, personal or family history of breast cancer, early age at menarche, late age at menopause, lengthy exposure to estrogen, never had children or late age at first live birth, and higher education and socioeconomic status. Variations in diet, especially fat intake, are currently being studied as a correlate to cancer incidence (American Cancer Society, 1995; Murphy et al., 1995). Breast cancer risk factors appear to be more useful in providing clues to the development of cancer than in identifying prevention strategies. Since African-American women may not be able to alter their personal risk factors in any practical sense, the best current opportunity for reducing mortality is through early detection (Murphy et al., 1995).

There are several methods of early detection recommended by the American Cancer Society and the National Cancer Institute (Murphy et al., 1995). It is recommended that asymptomatic women have a screening mammogram every one–two years; women age 50 and over should have a mammogram every year. In addition, a clinical physical examination of the breast is recommended every three years for women aged 20 to 40, and every year for those over 40. Monthly breast self-examination also is recommended as a routine good health habit for women 20 and older (American Cancer Society, 1995).

Researchers agree that early diagnosis and treatment are beneficial and that screening mammography can make an important contribution to early diagnosis (Baker, 1982; Shapiro et al., 1982; Tabar et al., 1985). Mammography is recognized as a valuable diagnostic technique for women who have findings suggestive of breast cancer. Mammography should, in theory, be available to all women. Despite some geographic maldistribution, there are more than enough mammography units in the United States to screen all of the age-eligible women (Brown et al., 1990). But whether the procedure is accessible to all women, particularly African-American women, at high risk of breast cancer is a critical question.

The cancer control supplement to the 1987 National Health Survey

(NHS) revealed disappointingly low use of screening mammography over-all. African-American women were less likely than Caucasians to undergo mammography (NCI Breast Cancer Screening Consortium, 1990). Low income and education and increasing age were also related to low use. In this survey significant proportions of the minority groups report never having heard of the test (Caplan et al., 1992).

Aside from early detection of breast cancer, there are treatment considerations should women be diagnosed with breast cancer. Taking into account the medical situation and the patient's preferences, treatment may require lumpectomy, mastectomy, radiation therapy, chemotherapy, or hormone manipulation therapy (American Cancer Society, 1995; Murphy et al., 1995).

Lung Cancer

Lung cancer is the most common site of cancer in both mortality and incidence, with an estimated 157,400 deaths and 169,900 new cases in 1995. In women a rapid increase, comparable to the increase observed in men in the 1940s (7 per 100,000 population in 1940 to 50 per 100,000 in 1990 for men) was seen starting in the mid-1960s (Murphy et al., 1992). Perhaps this reflects the fact that women began smoking cigarettes later than men did. In addition, women who started smoking in the 1940s were reaching ages 30 and 40 when cancer is more prevalent.

Lung cancer incidence is still increasing in women, although a decline was observed between the ages of 15 and 44. Incidence rates are slightly higher among African-American and Caucasian women (43.1 versus 40.2 per 100,000 persons) as seen in Table 5 (Miller et al., 1993). Overall, female mortality rates continue to increase, but at a slow rate. African-American and Caucasian women have similar rates of 29.4 and 29.8, respectively. Survival rates are poorer for African-American women compared to Caucasian women (13.0 versus 16.0 per 100,000 persons, respectively). Regardless of stage at diagnosis, the five-year relative survival rate is only 13% in all patients (Miller et al., 1993).

Cigarette smoking, exposure to certain industrial substances, and radiation exposure from occupational, medical, and environmental sources are known risk factors. Radon exposure, especially in cigarette smokers and sidestream smoking, also increases the risk for nonsmokers (American Cancer Society, 1995; Murphy et al., 1995).

Early detection of lung cancer can be difficult because symptoms often do not appear until the disease is in advanced stages. In smokers who stop smoking at the time of early precancerous cellular changes, damaged bronchial lining tissues often return to normal.

Chest X ray, analysis of types of cells contained in sputum, and fiber optic examination of the bronchial passages assist with diagnosis. Treat-

ment is determined by the type and stage of cancer. Options include surgery, radiation therapy, and chemotherapy, with surgery usually being the
treatment of choice (American Cancer Society, 1995; Murphy et al., 1995).

Colorectal Cancer

Incidence rates of colorectal cancer have increased since 1973 and a
decline was seen since 1985. Unfortunately, a significant decline was not
yet apparent among African-Americans (Miller et al., 1993). The incidence
rates increased for colorectal cancer for African-American women and a
decrease was seen among Caucasian women. From 1986 to 1990, the
overall rates for colorectal cancer were similar, but rates were 36 percent
higher for African-American women who were under 65 years of age than
for Caucasians in the same age group. National data showed that African-
American women experienced a higher rate than among Caucasian women
(46.8 versus 40.9 per 100,000 persons), as shown in Table 5 (Miller et al.,
1993).

Mortality from colorectal cancer increased significantly among African-
American women between 1973 to 1990 (i.e., 3.2 percent). Mortality decreased in African-American women aged 65 and older. Overall, mortality
rates were 20.6 and 16.0 for African-Americans and Caucasians, respectively (Miller et al., 1993).

The overall five-year survival for colon and rectal cancer is 56%. However, colon cancer five-year survival improves to 92% and rectal cancer to
85% when the disease is diagnosed at a localized stage (Murphy et al.,
1995). From 1983 to 1989, national data show that African-American
women had poorer survival rates compared to Caucasian women (48.9
versus 58.7 per 100,000 persons) (Miller et al., 1993).

Known predisposing conditions for colorectal cancer include personal
or family history of cancer or polyps of the colon or rectum and inflammatory bowel disease. High-fat and/or low-fiber diet also may be associated with increased risk.

Early detection of colorectal cancer is done through recommended
screening tests. Digital rectal examination, stool blood test, and proctosig-
moidoscopy are recommended to detect colon or rectum cancer in symp-
tomatic patients. Surgery, at times combined with radiation, is the most
effective method of treating colorectal cancer (American Cancer Society,
1955; Murphy et al., 1995).

Cervix Uteri

Incidence and mortality rates in African-American women continue to
decline in all age groups. While incidence rates for African-American
women over the age of 50 are still over twice those of Caucasian women,

the gap between African-American women under 50 is rapidly closing. According to Table 5, national data for African-American women show overall incidence rates of 14.3 per 100,000 persons compared to 7.9 for Caucasian women (Miller et al., 1993).

Mortality rates at all ages, however, continue to be much higher for African-American women. From 1986 to 1990, African-American women had mortality rates of 6.9 per 100,000 persons, while 2.6 was reported for Caucasian women (Miller et al., 1993).

African-American women under the age of 50 have experienced an unexplained 9 percentage-point decline in five-year relative survival for the most recent time period. Further investigation indicates that this decline is in cases initially diagnosed as a regional stage. The five-year survival rates for African-American women and Caucasian women were 57 and 69.1, respectively. The five-year survival rate for invasive cervical cancer is 67% overall, but 90% for cases diagnosed at an early stage. The survival for carcinoma in situ of the cervix is virtually 100% (Miller et al., 1993).

Known risk factors for cervix uteri are early age at first intercourse, multiple sex partners, cigarette smoking, and infections with certain types of human papillomavirus (American Cancer Society, 1995; Murphy et al., 1995). Much of the decline in rates has been associated with widespread use of the Pap test, which is a simple procedure that can be performed at appropriate intervals by health care professionals as part of a pelvic examination. This test should be performed annually with a pelvic examination in women who are, or have been, sexually active or who have reached 18. After three or more consecutive annual examinations with normal findings, the Pap test may be performed less frequently at the discretion of the physician (American Cancer Society, 1995).

Cervix cancers generally are treated by surgery or radiation, or by a combination of the two. In precancerous stages, changes in the cervix may be treated by cryotherapy, electrocoagulation, or local surgery (American Cancer Society, 1995; Murphy et al., 1995).

Cancer Control Efforts

A review of the burden of cancer among African-American women shows that mortality and incidence rates are higher and survival rates poorer compared to Caucasian women. These differences in rates suggest disparities among population segments and possible results of cancer control efforts. While survival rates for various cancers are improving for most patients, there are significant disparities among African-American women. This population segment appears to be exposed in greater proportion to the risk factors for cancer, especially the behavioral risks, to have cancer detected at an advanced stage, and to receive delayed treatment (Boring et al., 1992; Bal, 1992).

It appears that the trends in cancer among African-American women may represent myriad social, behavioral, environmental, economic, and educational factors. Statistical adjustment for income and education decrease the cancer rates for African-Americans below those of whites. However, the unfortunate fact remains that being an African-American correlates highly statistically significantly with being poor, less educated, and deprived of a healthy environment in which to live. Being an African-American becomes a convenient surrogate measure of these confounding factors and this seemingly increases one's risk of certain cancers (Murphy et al., 1995).

Suggested solutions for addressing problems of cancer among African-American women may include a risk-reduction program, focusing on nutrition and tobacco use, and improving availability, accessibility, and range of health care services, including screening and treatment. These solutions support a range of opportunities whereby the impact of cancer in African-American women can be diminished through cancer control efforts such as community programs and public health action.

CONCLUSIONS

Statistical data and general information for common cancer sites play an integral role in evaluating the scope of the cancer problem among African-American women and the results of cancer control efforts.

Clearly, cancer is a health issue for African-American women. What seems to be a health issue is in fact intertwined with social, behavioral, economic, and other concerns. Namely, African-American women's placement in the social structure in reference to health and illness, societal stereotypes about African-American women's health-related behavior, and the health status of these women are among important issues identified with emphasis on cancer. These issues call attention to social patterning of health being important to the size of the gap between the mortality and survival rates for population segments, giving some indication of the potential for improvement in African-American women's health. Identification of persons who are at greatest risk of poor health can inform sound governance of health and medical services. Further, the possible relationship between health and social position may suggest hypotheses concerning the etiology of common cancers among African-American women. Equally important, understanding the causes of social variations, societal labeling, and implications of health status should lead to intervention strategies that may reduce the burden of cancer.

Based on the discussion in this chapter, a number of areas can be identified that are important to future investigations. A more precise study about African-American women's placement in a social structure to explore social determinants of health would be useful. Investigations about the impact of slavery on the development of gynecologic cancers warrants attention, as does the examination of economic and social variations in relation to historical contexts. Further, studies should be directed toward understanding a combination of biological and psychosocial processes that impact the development of cancer in African-American women. While there may be various studies under way, there remains a great task for investigators who wish to conduct research for African-American women.

WORKS CITED

American Cancer Society (1989). *Cancer and the Poor: A Report to the Nation.* Atlanta: American Cancer Society.

American Cancer Society (1995). *American Cancer Facts and Figures.* Atlanta: American Cancer Society, 95, 375 M-No. 5008.95.

Baker, L. H. (1982). Breast cancer detection demonstration product: Five-Year Summary Report. *Cancer,* 32 (4), 194–225.

Bal, D. E. (1992). Cancer in African Americans. *Cancer Journal Clin,* 42 (1), 5–6.

Berkanovic, E. & Reeder, L. G. (1973). Ethnic, economic and social psychological factors in the source of medical care. *Social Problems,* 21, 246–259.

Blone, D. (1995). Social determinants of health-socioeconomic status, social class and ethnicity (editorial). *American Journal of Public Health,* 85, 903–905.

Boring, C. C., Squires, T. S. & Heath, C. W. (1992). *Cancer Statistics for African Americans.* Atlanta: American Cancer Society, 92-20M-N-3034-PE.

Brown, M. L., Kessler, L. G. & Reuter, F. G. (1990). Is the supply of mammography machines outstripping need and demand? An economic analysis. *American International Medicine,* 113, 547–552.

Caplan, L. S., Wells, B. L. & Haynes, S. (1992). Breast cancer screening among older racial/ethnic minorities and whites: barriers to early detection. *Journal of Gerontology,* 47, 101–110.

Childers, T. & Post, J. A. (1975). *The Information Poor in America.* Metuchen, NJ: Scarecrow Press.

Dervin, B. (1989). Audience as listener and learner, teacher and confidant: The sense making approach. In R. E. Rice & C. K. Atkin, eds., *Public Communication Companies,* 2nd ed. Newbury Park, CA.: Sage Publications.

Dodsom, J. (1981). Conceptualization of black families. In H. McAdoo, ed., *Black Families.* London: Sage Publications.

Feldman, J. (1966). *The Dissemination of Health Information.* Chicago: Aldine.

Freimuth, V. S. (1995). *Mass Media Strategies and Channels: A Review of the Use of Media in Breast and Cervical Cancers Screening Programs Wellness Perspectives: Research, Theory and Practice.* Atlanta: Centers for Disease Control and Prevention.

Freimuth, V. S., & Mettger W. (1990). Is There a Hard-to-Reach Audience? Public Health Report. 105(3) 232–238.

Harwood, A. (1981). *Ethnicity and Medical Care.* Cambridge, MA: Harvard University Press.

Henderson, G. P. & Primeaux, M. (1981). *Transcultural Health Care.* Menlo Park,

CA.: Addison-Wesley.

Holmes, T. H. & Rohe, R. H. (1967). The social readjustment scale. *Journal of Psychosomatic Research,* 11 (2), 213–218.

Insel, P. M. & Moos, R. H. (1994). *Health in the Social Environment.* Lexington, MA: D. C. Heath.

Institute of Medicine. (1985). *Preventing Low Birth Weight.* Washington, DC.: National Academy Press.

Levine, S. & Scotch, N. A. (1970). *Social Stress.* Chicago: Aldine.

Lyons, J. (1972). Methods of successful communication with the disadvantaged. In *Communication for Change with the Rural Disadvantaged.* Washington, DC: National Academy of Sciences.

McKnight, J. L. (1985). Where can health communication be found? Presented at the International Communication Association Convention, Honolulu.

Mechanic, D. (1989). Socioeconomic status and health: An examination of underlying processes. In J. P. Bunker, D. S. Goinby, & B. H. Kehrer, eds., *Pathways to Health: The Role of Social Factors.* Menlo Park, CA: Henry J. Kaiser Foundation.

Miller, B. A., Ries, L. A. G., Honkey, B. F. et al. (1993). *SEER Cancer Statistics Review 1973–1990.* Bethesda, MD: National Cancer Institute, NIH Publication No. 93-2789.

Murphy, G. P., Lawrence, W. & Lenhard, R. E. (1995). *Clinical Oncology,* 2nd ed. Atlanta: American Cancer Society.

Myrdal, G. (1944). *An American Dilemma: The Negro Problem of Modern Democracy.* New York: Harper & Bros.

National Academy of Science. (1984). *Report of the Panel on Decennial Census Methodology.* Committee on National Statistics, National Research Council. Washington, DC: National Academy Press.

National Center for Health Statistics. (1992). *Health, United States 1992.* Hyattsville, MD: National Center for Health Statistics, DHHS Publication No. (PHS)93-1232.

NCI Breast Cancer Screening Consortium. (1990). Screening mammography: A misused clinical opportunity? Results of the NCI Breast Cancer Screening Consortium and National Health Interview Survey Studies. *JAMA,* 264, 54–58.

O'Hara, W. P., Pollard, K. M., Mann, T. L. & Kent, M. M. (1991). African Americans in the 1990s. *Population Bulletin,* 46 (1), 2–40.

Olesen, V. (1977). *Women and Their Health: Research Implications for a New Era.* Springfield, VA: National Technical Information Service.

Reed, W. L., Darity, W. & Roberson, N. L. (1993). *Health and Medical Care of African Americans.* Westport, CT.: Auburn House.

Schatzman, L. & Strauss, A. (1955). Social class and modes of communication. *American Journal of Sociology,* 60, 329–338.

Schreiber, J. M. & Homiak, J. P. (1981). Mexican Americans. In A. Harwood, ed., *Ethnicity and Medical Care.* Cambridge, MA: Harvard University Press.

Smith, W. C. (1985). *The Church in the Life of the Black Family.* Valley Forge, PA.: Judson Press.

Sorlie, P. D., Backlund, E. & Keller, J. B. (1995). U.S. mortality by economic, demographic and social characteristics: The National Longitudinal Mortality Study. *American Journal of Public Health*, 85, 949–956.

Shapiro, S., Strax, P., Venet, L. & Rosen, R. (1982). Ten-to-fourteen years' effect of screening on breast cancer mortality. *Journal of National Cancer Institute*, 69, 349–353.

Suchman, E. A. (1964). Sociomedical variations among ethnic groups. *American Journal of Sociology*, 70, 319–331.

Suderkasa, N. (1981). Interpreting the Afro-American heritage in the Afro-American family organization. In H. McAdoo, ed., *Black Families*. London: Sage Publications.

Tabar, L., Gad. A., Holmquist, U. et al. (1985). Reduction from breast cancer after mass screening with mammography. Randomized trial from the Breast Cancer Working Group of the Swedish National Board of Health and Welfare. *Lancet* 8433, 829–832.

U.S. Bureau of the Census (1992). The black population in the United States, March 1991. *Current Population Reports*, Series P-20, No. 464. Washington, DC: U.S.Government Printing Office.

U.S. Bureau of the Census (1993). *We the American Blacks*. Washington, DC: U.S. Government Printing Office.

U.S. Department of Health and Human Services. (1985). Office of the Secretary. *Report of the Secretary's Task Force on Black and Minority Health*. Executive Summary, vol. 1. Washington, DC.

U.S. Department of Health and Human Services. (1990). *Minority Aging: Essential Curricula Content for Selected Health and Allied Health Professionals*. Washington, DC: Public Health Services, 193–321. Publication No. HRS-P-DV 90-4.

U.S. Department of Health and Human Services. (1994a). *Chronic Disease in Minority Population: African Americans, American Indians and Alaska Natives, Asians and Pacific Islanders, Hispanic Americans*. Atlanta: Centers for Disease Control and Prevention.

U.S. Department of Health and Human Services. (1994b). *Healthy People: National Health Promotion and Disease Prevention Objectives*. Washington, DC: U.S. Government Printing Office.

Water, M. C. (1991). The role of lineage in identity formation among black Americans. *Qualitative Social*, 14 (1) 57–76.

4

Hypertension and African-American Women

Cynthia Crawford-Green

Hypertension is an extremely common malady within the African-American community. It wreaks its havoc indiscriminately: across elusive socio-economic lines, educational attainment, profession, or region of the country. As women of color have made impressive strides toward equality in the workplace, so too has the morbidity and mortality of cardiovascular disease shown an upward spiral. For too long hypertension has been the "silent killer" of American blacks. The reasons are not subtle. Unfortunately the disease plays a very cruel hoax upon its victims. Time and time again patients remark that they feel fine—"I just have a little 'pressure' "— only to be struck down in the prime of life with a debilitating or fatal cerebrovascular accident or stroke. The data are clear that control of blood pressure can reduce the incidence of stroke; but, again, many patients are unable to achieve that control for a variety of reasons, including but not limited to: lack of access to a health care provider, inability to afford the medications, intolerable side effects of medications, lack of close follow-up by the treating physician and inattention to inadequately controlled blood pressure, obesity, smoking, and *stress.*

An important but often overlooked critical factor is that hypertension is a multisystem disease—it negatively affects the heart, blood vessels, brain, liver, lungs, eyes, and kidneys. So an inattention to proper control of the blood pressure can have far-reaching and unsuspected clinical implications. Treating physicians want the blood pressure to be normal when it is checked during an office visit. However, if salt and caloric intake are modified or the medications are taken only two to three days before the visit in order for the "pressure to be down" at that time, those efforts are sadly misguided, for the end organ damage caused by uncontrolled blood pressure marches inexorably silently on while this charade with no winners is played out.

In this chapter I will briefly provide an overview of hypertension and its impact on African-American women. I will not attempt to provide all of the answers to the pressing questions that will be raised; however, it is my hope that this will be a springboard for those interested and inspired readers to assist in the monumental task of fashioning an ethnically and gender-specific response to this serious public health care concern.

DEFINITION

Blood pressure is a continuous dynamic variable—meaning that it is normal expected physiology for the blood pressure to change with different levels of physical or mental exertion or time of the day or season of the year. Three large cross-sectional studies, the National Health and Nutrition Examination Surveys, (NHANES), were carried out in the United States between 1960 and 1962, 1971 and 1974, and 1976 and 1980. Based on the data from the 1976–1980 study, estimates of 57.7 million people with hypertension (a reading of 160/95) according to the 1960–1962 study findings, the number had more than doubled. Subsequently, however, many studies clearly demonstrated that the risk for cardiovascular diseases progressively rises with systolic blood pressure levels over 140 and diastolic blood pressure levels greater than 90. This change to a lower diagnostic criterion as well as more elderly persons resulted in the apparent explosion in the number of Americans affected with hypertension (Dannenberg et al., 1987; Joint National Committee, 1985). Indeed, in the United States hypertension has become the most frequent reason for doctor visits and prescription medications (Gross et al., 1989; Persky et al., 1986). For the most accurate definition of hypertension, an elevated blood pressure should be recorded on at least three separate occasions in the appropriate clinical environment—in the supine position in a quiet warm setting. This caution is warranted because the "white coat" phenomenon is frequently observed when the patient is anxious at the time of the initial blood pressure recording by the physician. If, however, the patient is allowed to relax and he or she feels comfortable with the physician, then the blood pressure frequently will return to lower or even normal levels. This is not a small point, as many asymptomatic individuals with only minimally elevated blood pressures may be inappropriately treated, resulting in the cost of therapy as well as the potential of adverse side effects. Ambulatory blood pressure readings or out-of-office recordings have varied 22/12 mm Hg from readings obtained in the office (Saito et al., 1990). It is likely, therefore, that these readings may become more widely used clinically in both the diagnosis and therapy of systemic hypertension.

If blood pressure recordings are consistently greater than 140/90, the diagnosis of hypertension is certain. The following list shows the classification of hypertension as defined by the 1988 Joint National Committee on the Detection, Evaluation and Treatment of High Blood Pressure (p. 1023):

Diastolic Blood Pressure

<85	Normal Blood Pressure
85–89	High-normal Blood Pressure
90–104	Mild hypertension
105–114	Moderate hypertension
>/115	Severe hypertension

Systolic BP when Diastolic BP <90

<140	Normal Blood Pressure
140–159	Borderline systolic isolated hypertension
>/160	Isolated systolic hypertension

CAUSES

The vast majority of affected individuals have essential or primary hypertension. The etiology is felt to be multifactorial, including genetic, hormonal, neurogenic, and vascular components (Joint National Committee, 1988; Perloff, 1989; Oparil, 1988; Kaplan, 1992; Hildreth & Saunders, 1991). There are, however, many secondary causes of hypertension. Renal disease may lead directly to hypertension, even though among blacks it is far more common for hypertension to result in renal failure. Some renal causes include glomerulonephritis, interstitial nephritis, polycystic kidney, systemic lupus erythematosus, and renal artery occlusive disease. Interestingly, SLE, and its resultant hypertension, are not uncommon among black women, but fibromuscular dysplasia which results in abnormal narrowing of the renal arteries is overwhelmingly observed in young white women. Less common endocrine or glandular causes are acromegaly, Cushing's disease, pheochromocytoma, hyperthyroidism (overactive thyroid gland), and hypothyroidism (underactive thyroid gland). A congenital narrowing of the aorta called coarctation of the aorta is another uncommon secondary cause of hypertension. It often can be diagnosed in childhood and the treatment is surgical repair. Checking the blood pressure in both arms is a quick and easy method to rule out this disorder.

Pregnancy-induced hypertension is a very common secondary cause of hypertension. Normally, during pregnancy the blood pressure should decrease even to levels slightly lower than the baseline readings obtained before pregnancy. In fact, among gravid women, a blood pressure of 140/90, which defines mild hypertension otherwise, is considered severe hypertension. Preeclampsia unfortunately is commonly observed among black patients, especially younger first-time mothers often of lower socioeconomic status. Preeclampsia or toxemia of pregnancy is characterized by hypertension, headache, right upper quadrant pain, and edema of the feet, legs, and hands. If left untreated, preeclampsia may result in low-birth-weight infants, seizures, renal failure, and death of either the mother or the baby. Preeclampsia does not usually occur in subsequent pregnancies, but it may. Less dramatically, blood pressure elevations in the absence of the other features of toxemia may occur in pregnancy. In both settings, the blood pressure usually returns to normal levels after the delivery of the baby. It is felt that mothers who develop hypertension during pregnancy may be more likely to develop systemic hypertension at some point later in life (James & Healy, 1989; Drayer & Zegarelli, 1989).

Neurological causes of hypertension include increased intracranial pressure, which may result after head trauma, stroke or mass effect, tumor, sleep apnea, lead poisoning, and quadriplegia. During acute stress the blood pressure may rise and this phenomenon is observed in several clinical settings including surgery, alcohol or illicit drug ingestion, alcohol withdrawal syndrome (delirium tremens, or DTs), sickle-cell crisis, burns, pancreatitis, and hypoglycemia. The secondary causes of hypertension are many and the items listed herein are not exclusive. The treatment of this secondary hypertension is usually directed at the underlying cause (Oparil, 1988).

PREVALENCE

Among all women ages 18 to 74, 25.3% of white women have hypertension compared to 38.6% of black women (Perloff, 1989; Haywood, 1990). As you can see from Table 6, at every age black women have more hypertension than their white counterparts.

After the age of 40 the difference becomes quite striking. Although data clearly demonstrate that hypertension is very common in black women and nearly ubiquitous in some age groups, the reason or reasons are not clearly defined. Clearly, obesity and stress play a role, but they are not the whole answer. Elucidation of these enigmatic factors may eventually lead to the fashioning of effective strategies for prevention, treatment, and cure.

Hypertension is more commonly observed in blacks compared to

**Table 6
Age-Specific Hypertension
Prevalence Among Black and
White Women**

Age	Percentage White vs. Black
18 to 24	2.3 vs. 9.6
25 to 34	5.7 vs. 15.3
35 to 44	16.6 vs. 37.0
45 to 54	6.3 vs. 67.0
55 to 64	50.0 vs. 74.3
65 to 74	66.2 vs. 82.9

whites, and it is also more severe (Joint National Committee, 1988; Hildreth & Saunders, 1991; Haywood, 1990). The NHANES 1971–1974 survey revealed that among all black and white women enrollees aged 18 to 74, a normal blood pressure was recorded in 73.3% of whites and 62.9% of blacks. Mild hypertension was seen in 10.8% of whites and 17.9% of blacks, moderate hypertension in 1.1% of whites and 3.1% of blacks, and severe hypertension in 0.4% of whites and 0.8% of blacks.

MEDICAL HISTORY

Most women will have essential or idiopathic hypertension, which is overwhelmingly the most common form among all ethnic and gender groups. Each patient should, however, be completely evaluated in order to exclude other causes and to determine the presence, if any, of end organ damage. Initially each woman should undergo a complete history and physical examination. The health care provider should ask a large number of questions that at first glance may appear unrelated to the diagnosis of hypertension. First, one must elucidate the symptoms. As hypertension is also called the silent killer, the examiner must be sensitive to the observation that most patients will initially deny any problems. Upon closer examination, however, one may elicit a history of fatigue, malaise, headache, blurred vision, sleeplessness, weight gain, palpitations, chest tightness, and so on. The woman may have noticed that these vague nonspecific symptoms have gradually appeared over several months to years. Oftentimes the symptoms may be attributed to stress or getting older. Of course these findings are neither unique to nor diagnostic of hypertension. As hypertension can primarily affect the cardiovascular system, a careful cardiac history must be performed. One should be asked about the presence of palpitations or heart fluttering in the chest or skipping beats, chest pain that may be described as heaviness, pressure, sharp, or burning with exertion. Dyspnea or difficulty breathing may also accompany the chest discomfort. Claudication may be described as a pain, numbness, or cramping in the calves of the legs with exertion that is related to reduced blood flow to the muscles. Numbness or tingling in any part of the body may signal a stroke or neurological damage, and this is certainly seen in hypertension and is probably the most dreaded complication because of the devastating potential. Blood in the urine while not menstruating (hematuria) may signal kidney damage (Perloff, 1989; Oparil, 1988; Kaplan, 1992).

In addition to discussing the symptoms, a thorough past medical history and family history should be obtained. In other words, has the patient ever been told at any time that she had an elevated blood pressure. Determine when she was told and what therapy, if any, was instituted. Also the response to therapy is crucial. Many patients will say "I was told once that I had hypertension but it went away and I no longer take medicine for it." It is the unusual patient, however, who was removed from the medical regimen by her health care provider! Not uncommonly, patients feel better after the blood pressure has been controlled for a while and they erroneously assume that the high blood pressure has been cured. Alternatively, the blood pressure readings are normal in the office and the patient again assumes that she is cured. What she has failed to realize, however, is that the blood pressure is normal because of the medical regimen, weight loss, and exercise that are working in concert to control the blood pressure, but the hypertension cannot be cured. Hypertension is felt to have a strong genetic component; thus it is essential to determine the presence of hypertension in parents, siblings, and other relatives. If all family members develop hypertension by the age of 35 and require multiple medications, it is very likely that your patient will have a similar history. As we have mentioned, it is generally recommended that it requires multiple readings at different settings in order to diagnose hypertension. When a significant family history is added to a patient with minimally elevated blood pressure, some health care providers would be much more likely to initiate therapy. It is important also to elicit a history of factors that contribute to the development of hypertension, including smoking, excessive alcohol ingestion, oral contraceptive use, diabetes mellitus, excessive salt intake, and illicit drug use (Perloff, 1989; Oparil, 1988; Kaplan, 1992).

It is important to determine if the affected family members have heart disease or renal disease. In this country the most common cause of end-stage renal disease requiring dialysis unfortunately is hypertension. There are multiple research studies ongoing to determine if very good control of the blood pressure can prevent or delay the onset of renal disease. This is a very important point because even though blacks make up the majority of the dialysis patients in certain parts of this country, only a minority of renal transplantations in this country are performed on blacks.

SOCIAL HISTORY

One cannot adequately treat a black woman with hypertension without obtaining a complete social and work history. There is no doubt that job stress is a major contributing factor to the development of hypertension. Studies using ambulatory blood pressure monitoring have clearly shown that the blood pressure increases during the day at work and during commuting times. Often when the patient is in a calmer environment the blood pressure will greatly improve. While on the job, the patient should be counseled regarding relaxation, time out, and other stress-reduction mechanisms. It is important to alert the patient that only a finite amount of work can be accomplished daily even by the most dynamic superwoman. If she has worked diligently on the assigned tasks and remains continuously overwhelmed, she should know that it is okay to talk openly and honestly with her supervisors regarding restructuring her duties to a more reasonable level. In this era of corporate downsizing, reinventing government with massive layoffs, and exporting jobs to cheaper countries, many women (and men) are rightly concerned about maintaining their employment. One should not, however, literally work one's self to death. It is also crucial to realize that these pressures are very common; therefore the specifics of the work environment should not be pursued only among the white-collar professionals. Despite the best efforts of all involved, there will be occasions where extended leave, transfer to another position, or leaving the workplace altogether will be recommended.

In addition to the workplace, many women of color face another battleground when they return home. It is a sad and sobering fact that many women return to a home where they are the head of the household. They serve as the sole provider for themselves, their children, their grandchildren, and other extended family members as needs arise. Owing to the very young age that many women begin to bear children, it is not unusual for women to be great-grandmothers before reaching age 50. The frustrations grow as many women view the prime years of their lives being complicated by yet another set of children for whom there are inadequate resources and levels of support.

In my practice setting in Washington, D.C., it is numbing when I recount the number of my patients who have sons, daughters, and grandchildren who have succumbed to the lure of the streets as evidenced by illicit drug abuse, retailing of illicit drugs, and other criminal activities that resulted in tragic early deaths. It is more than once that I have been dismayed that a patient's blood pressure is totally out of control compared to the previous levels. When I question her I'm told "Well, another one of my grandchildren was shot down in the street last night just like a dog." Or when asking the women in my practice about their children, it also is unbelievable that 30 to 40% of the women have children locked up in city, state, and federal institutions. These women often are consumed with the notion of retrieving their sons from this incarceration, but they lack the money and the connections most often required to accomplish this goal. They mourn at birthdays that can't be shared; they cry when they can't help all of the grandchildren sired by their sons by several different women; they are at a loss to care for their daughters' children by multiple absent noncontributing fathers.

These are not the ramblings of a right-wing zealot. Instead they represent the reality of inner-city medicine. These social ills have crept into suburbia and the countryside as well. Unless and until there is a dramatic change in these harsh realities, one can only anticipate that stress-induced and stress-exacerbated hypertension will persist. The health care provider may not have all of the answers to change the lives of many patients; however, it is uplifting to some to know that you cared enough to ask about it and demonstrated genuine concern.

As stated above, often women in the black community are the sole breadwinner in the family, and, as we know, black women's salaries are not comparable to white women with the same educational and experience backgrounds. The salaries of black men are well below those of white men with similar backgrounds; so for many black couples working hard and striving to succeed, it has become increasingly difficult to make the proverbial ends meet. For all of these reasons, black women are asked to make bricks without straw on a daily basis. When money is a premium, it is not at all unusual for patients to bypass the purchase of their medicine in order to pay for other necessities, such as food, shelter, and transportation.

The elderly patient is particularly vulnerable. With reduction in social payments, it is harder for retirees to supplement their incomes with Medicaid or welfare payments. As a result, the cost of the medicines is often out of reach for many because Medicare covers the cost of office, hospital, and doctor visits at 80% of the allowed amount; but it does not cover the cost of any medications. One, therefore, must ask if the patient is no longer taking the drug because she simply cannot afford it. Neither the health care provider nor the patient should be shy when addressing these very real fiscal concerns. Worsening and progression of the disease, hospitalization, and death may needlessly occur because the patient had no medication.

For women who work but do not carry health insurance the story is the same. It is incumbent upon the physician to encourage all of his or her patients to obtain health insurance if at all possible. Even though the cost may seem high to some on a tight budget, it must be shown that not to have coverage is to be penny-wise but pound-foolish. There are some pharmaceutical companies that either provide drugs for indigent patients or pay the cost of any additional medication if their drug does not adequately control the blood pressure alone. Also, physicians receive sample medications that can be used to supplement the prescriptions of patients. A combination of these and other creative methods may be required to assure that the patient has an adequate supply of medicine.

PHYSICAL EXAMINATION

The physical examination of a woman with hypertension should be directed to confirm the diagnosis and to detect the presence of end organ damage. First, the blood pressure should be taken in both arms, ideally when the patient is lying, sitting, and standing. Recording of height and weight are important because hypertension is associated with obesity. Examination of the head should include palpation and auscultation of the carotid arteries. Fundoscopic examination of the fundus will reveal the signs of hypertensive retinopathy. There are changes in the eyes that generally accompany long-standing hypertension. Grade 1 changes are silver wiring or mild narrowing of the arteries. Grade 2 changes include more pronounced narrowing of the arteries, grade 3 changes include marked narrowing of the arteries with hemorrhages and exudates in the fundus, and finally grade 4 changes (which are the most severe) include papilledema or swelling of the fundus along with the hemorrhages and exudates. Grade 4 changes represent a medical emergency, and prompt hospitalization in an intensive care unit with rapid lowering of the blood pressure are indicated (Oparil, 1988; Kaplan, 1992; Fox & Shapiro, 1986).

All peripheral pulses should be checked in order to determine the presence of significant occlusive disease that may be evidenced by diminished pulses, bruits, or thrills. The examination of the heart includes palpation of the left ventricular apex in order to determine if left ventricular hypertrophy is present. When one feels the apex of the heart it may be forceful and prolonged, suggesting that the heart muscle is thickened. When one listens to the heart, one listens for an extra sound called an S4 gallop, which also usually accompanies long-standing hypertension. The remainder of the cardiac examination will be directed at excluding valvular abnormalities that may contribute to hypertension, such as aortic stenosis. Also congestive heart failure can be excluded if no S3 gallop or fluid in the lungs is appreciated. The abdomen must be examined for abnormal sounds from the arteries called bruits, and finally a careful neurological examination is needed in order to rule out any stigmata of a stroke (Perloff, 1989; Oparil, 1988; Hildreth & Saunders, 1991).

LABORATORY TESTS

Blood tests that would be performed as part of the routine medical evaluation should be done as an initial evaluation of the hypertensive patient. These include hemoglobin and hematocrit, creatinine, blood urea nitrogen, electrolytes, and urinalysis. As most of these tests are now available on an automated panel at a lower cost than individual tests, other studies would also routinely be obtained including blood glucose, serum cholesterol, uric acid, calcium, and liver enzymes. A baseline electrocardiogram is required and controversy exists regarding the necessity of obtaining an echocardiogram on every hypertensive patient. It is usual practice, however, that an echocardiogram (sound wave picture of the heart made by the same method to view the baby in a pregnant woman) will be performed at some time during the treatment of the hypertensive patient in an effort to visualize left ventricular function and hypertrophy. Chest X rays are probably not as universally done now as in previous years. If these studies are normal, they need not be repeated more frequently than once per year unless symptoms dictate otherwise.

THERAPY

The goal of therapeutic intervention in hypertension is to reduce the excess cardiovascular morbidity and mortality. As noted above, the decision to initiate therapy is guided by the degree of blood pressure elevation and the presence of end organ damage. Therapy is usually started in patients with diastolic blood pressures in excess of 95 mm Hg. Patients with lesser diastolic blood pressures of 90 to 94 mm Hg may have therapy if there is an increased risk for cardiovascular complications, including those with involvement of kidney, diabetes, hyperlipidemia, or history of a heart attack (Joint National Committee, 1988; Perloff, 1989; Oparil, 1988; Hildreth & Saunders, 1991).

Nonpharmacologic therapy is usually the first line in patients with only minimally elevated blood pressures without evidence of end organ damage. Dietary sodium (salt) restriction is the most effective of the nonpharmacologic measures. Moderate salt restriction (4 to 6 grams per day) lowers blood pressure and helps the antihypertensive effects of diuretics. On the other hand, a high sodium intake of 15 to 20 grams per day may overcome the antihypertensive effect of diuretics. Patients should be counseled about the high sodium content in processed foods. I strive to have patients add only a small amount of salt to food during cooking and none at the table. Salt substitute preparations can also be used in moderation. The reduction of salt in the diet is very important in the care of the hypertensive at all stages, and it is incumbent upon the health care provider to remind the patient at frequent intervals. Also, patients should be told that the food can have soul and can have taste without the large amount of salt that traditionally many black and Southern cooks have used.

Weight loss is an important part of the regimen as a large percentage of black women are overweight. Some studies have shown that over 50% of women over the age of 45 are overweight. Reduction of weight can lead to a reduction in the blood pressure. Patients should be told that it is likely that they will require less medication if they can achieve an ideal body weight. It rarely occurs that no further medication may be necessary. Weight loss is achieved not by spending thousands of dollars at franchised weight-loss facilities, for miracle pills or herbs, or for the most advanced fat-burning exercise equipment. The secret of weight loss that these entrepreneurs have capitalized upon and packaged for public consumption is as follows: (1) *eat less,* (2) *exercise more.*

There are no other ways to achieve successful sustained weight loss. It is not easy and the road at times may seem interminable. However, with the loss of the first pound, one can readily see that it is possible. Patients must be counseled that the weight did not get there quickly and it will not leave quickly. It also is important to teach black women that there are alternative cooking methods, including baking, broiling, and boiling. There are vegetables that can be well-prepared without large amounts of salted meats. Herbs and spices exist that can yield interesting flavor, and one should not be limited to the familiar tang of salt only. I stress to patients that they need not join the most expensive spa in town or buy the latest exercise equipment. On the contrary, a consistent exercise pattern that begins slowly but is maintained at an acceptable pace is far more effective than two hours of aerobics once every six months! Finally, weight loss will not only improve hypertension but it will improve glucose tolerance as well. The most common type of diabetes in black women is Type II, which is overwhelmingly associated with obesity. Improved glucose control can be observed among diabetic patients who are able to lose weight. Stress reduction and relaxation techniques are other less-well-documented measures used to improve blood pressure control.

MEDICAL THERAPY

If nonpharmacologic measures are ineffective for lowering the blood pressure, then medical therapy must be instituted. There are many drugs available for the treatment of hypertension today and the choice of drug is individualized by the physician for the patient. Previously the prescribing practices were much more dogmatic: start with a diuretic; increase drugs to the maximum tolerable dose. The goal today is to fashion a medical regimen for a patient that is effective, easy to take, has few side effects, and is affordable. There are many drug preparations available today that require only once-daily dosing, and ideally the initial drug should be chosen from this group. A drug should be given a reasonable amount of time before reevaluation is performed, usually one to four weeks in the mild to moderate hypertensive.

Among patients with severe hypertension, the response to therapy should probably be checked within two weeks. If the blood pressure partially responds to a drug in adequate doses, a second or third drug may be added in stages. There are occasions when a severe hypertensive patient is started on therapy and the initial regimen will consist of two to three drugs. This is not the practice for the usual patient; but in some in whom the blood pressure is markedly elevated, there is little concern that the medication will reduce the pressure too quickly or too low (Saito et al., 1990; Perloff, 1989; Oparil, 1988; Kaplan, 1992).

There are several classes of drugs available and they include diuretics, beta blockers, central acting adrenergic inhibitors, peripheral acting adrenergic inhibitors, alphal-adrenergic blockers, vasodilators, angiotensin converting enzyme inhibitors, and calcium channel blockers. Diuretics are also known as water pills and they increase urination to rid the body of excess volume and thereby lower the blood pressure. Diuretics are often the first drug given to patients but with the entry into the market of other drug classes, many physicians reserve diuretics for volume reduction only—that is, swollen ankles and hands. Several years ago the MRFIT (multiple risk factors intervention trial) study demonstrated increased mortality among patients receiving diuretics. It is now felt that that was likely due to diuretic induced hypokalemia (low potassium), which increases the likelihood of developing arrhythmias. Other side effects associated with diuretics include hyperuricemia, glucose intolerance, hypercholesterolemia, hypertriglyceridemia, and sexual dysfunction. Some diuretic trade names include Lasix, HCTZ, Lozol, and Zaroxylyn (Oparil, 1988; Kaplan, 1992).

Controversy existed for several years regarding the use of beta blockers in black patients. Studies suggested that blacks did not respond well to the drug, but the current thinking is that black patients will respond but many will require higher doses. Side effects of beta blockers include bradycardia (slow heart rate), fatigue, insomnia, strange dreams, sexual dysfunction, decreased high-density lipoprotein cholesterol (good cholesterol). These drugs should be avoided in patients with asthma, chronic obstructive pulmonary disease, diabetes mellitus, congestive heart failure, and sick sinus syndrome. Some trade names of beta blockers include Inderal, Lopressor, Tenormin, and Corgard (Oparil, 1988; Kaplan, 1992).

Central acting drugs most commonly used today are Aldomet and Catapres. Common side effects include drowsiness, dry mouth, fatigue, and sexual dysfunction. Catapress may cause severe rebound hypertension if the drug is abruptly stopped. For that reason, it should be used by reliable patients. There is also a patch placed on the skin that must be changed only once per week. This has improved compliance and reduced the worst side effects for this drug. Aldomet is an older drug that should be taken two to four times daily. It is commonly used in the hypertensive pregnant woman because it has a favorable side effect profile among these patients (Oparil, 1988; Kaplan, 1992).

Minipress is the alphal-adrenergic blocking agent. It can cause first-dose syncope (passing out). It is therefore recommended that dosing be done at bedtime and it should be avoided in the elderly patient because of orthostatic hypotension. Labetolol is a combined alpha and beta blocker that can cause asthma, nausea, fatigue, dizziness, and headache. It is contraindicated in patients with heart failure, heart block greater than first degree, asthma, and chronic obstructive pulmonary disease.

Vasodilators include Apresoline and Loniten. Apresoline can cause a positive antinuclear antibody test and it may cause a lupus syndrome in larger doses. Loniten is a powerful antihypertensive that is reserved for the severe resistant hypertensive. The most common side effects include excessive hair growth and marked peripheral edema. This drug must be used with a diuretic. In the initial clinical studies the excess facial and body hair were noted. Further study of the drug was done and reformulation to a topical form produced the drug used for male pattern baldness called Rogaine! (Oparil, 1988; Kaplan, 1992). Angiotensin-converting enzymes include Capoten, Prinivil, Zestril, Accupril, and Vasotec. These drugs can cause a chronic cough and rash. Rarely they have been associated with abrupt swelling of the epiglottis. Acute renal failure, neutropenia, and proteinuria may occur as well. These drugs are commonly used in the treatment of hypertension among patients with diabetes mellitus because it appears that their use can delay the progression of diabetic nephropathy. ACE inhibitors are also frequently used in heart failure and after myocardial infarctions. Thus, this is a useful drug class because more than one problem can be treated with a single drug with a relatively benign side effect profile.

Finally, calcium channel blockers are a highly effective class of drugs. The most common ones include Calan, Verelan, Isoptin, Procardia, and Cardizem. These drugs are also effective in the treatment of chest-pain syndromes and hypertrophic cardiomyopathy where they have been shown to improve left ventricular diastolic function. These drugs are useful in the hypertensive patient for that same reason. Side effects include constipation, flushing, and peripheral edema. Recently these drugs have come under intense scrutiny after reports that there was increased mortality observed among patients taking them. That study resulted in a huge amount of press coverage and many panic-stricken patients stopped taking the drug unnecessarily. It is accepted that there is probably no role for the calcium channel blockers in the acute myocardial infarction setting, but it is an effective drug for the treatment of mild to severe hypertension. Additional studies are under way to fully characterize the effect of calcium channel blockers to the increased morbidity and mortality among patients with coronary artery disease (Oparil, 1988; Kaplan, 1992; Hildreth & Saunders, 1991).

CONCLUSION

Black women have hypertension much more frequently than white women and it is also much more severe. The cause of hypertension is unknown but there is no doubt that genetics, obesity, and stress along with humoral and cellular mechanisms play contributing complex roles in the pathogenesis of hypertension. Black women also tend to have more side effects related to hypertension. The treatment should be multifaceted and the nonpharmacological therapeutic modalities cannot be overlooked or minimized in importance. Medical therapy is important in order to avoid or delay the end organ damage associated with hypertension and that disproportionately affects black women, including eye disease, heart disease, heart failure, kidney disease, and stroke. The cost of medicine is high and many black women are unable to afford their medical regimen. Health care providers must continue to fashion innovative strategies for the care of these patients in order to avoid premature death and disability. Finally, we cannot attack this multisystem disease without a concerted effort to confront the ills of society that contribute directly and inexorably to the magnitude of this epidemic.

WORKS CITED

Dannenberg, A. L., Drizd, T. & Horan, M. J. et al. (1987). Progress in the battle against hypertension: Changes in blood pressure levels in the United States from 1960 to 1980. *Hypertension,* 10, 226.

Drayer, J. & Zegarelli, E. (1989). Hypertension and pregnancy. In P. Douglas, ed., *Heart Disease in Women.* Philadelphia: F. A. Davis Company.

Fox, K. & Shapiro, L. (1986). *Color Atlas of Hypertension.* London: Wolfe Medical Publisher, distributor for Year Book Medical Publishers.

Gross, T. P., Wise, R. P. & Knapp, D. E. (1989). Antihypertensive drug use: Trends in the United States from 1973 to 1985. *Hypertension* (Suppl. I).

Haywood, L. J. (1990). Hypertension in minority populations: Access to care. *American Journal of Medicine,* 88, 17S–20S.

Hildreth, C. & Saunders, E. (1991). Hypertension in blacks: Clinical overview. In Elijah Saunders, ed., *Cardiovascular Disease in Blacks.* Philadelphia: F. A. Davis Company.

James, K. & Healy, B. (1989). Heart disease arising during or secondary to pregnancy. In P. Douglas, ed., *Heart Disease in Women.* Philadelphia: F. A. Davis Company.

Joint National Committee. (1985). Subcommittee on Definition and Prevalence of the 1984 JNC. Hypertension prevalence and the status of awareness, treatment and control in the U.S. *Hypertension,* 7, 641.

Joint National Committee on the Detection, Evaluation and Treatment of High Blood Pressure (1985 & 1988). *Archives of Internal Medicine.*

Kaplan, N. (1992). Systemic hypertension: Mechanisms and diagnosis. In Eugene Braunwald, ed., *Heart Disease: A Textbook of Cardiovascular Medicine,* 4th ed. Philadelphia: W. B. Saunders.

Oparil, S. (1988). Arterial hypertension. In James B. Wyngraarden and Lloyd Smith, eds., *Cecil Textbook of Medicine,* 18th ed. Philadelphia: W. B. Saunders.

Perloff, D. (1989). Hypertension in women. In P. Douglas, ed., *Heart Disease in Women.* Philadelphia: F. A. Davis Company.

Persky, V., Pan, W. H., Stamler, J. et al. (1986). Time trends in the United States racial differences in hypertension. *American Journal of Epidemiology,* 124, 724–737.

Saito, I., Takeshita, E., Hayashi, S. et al. (1990). Comparison of clinic and home blood pressure levels and the role of the sympathetic nervous system in clinic-home differences. *American Journal of Hypertension,* 3, 219.

5

Focus on African-American Women and Diabetes

Catherine Fisher Collins

Diabetes is a disease that is ravishing the African-American community. Some estimate that there are 10 million Americans "with some form of diabetes, and half of those do not know that they have it" (Edlin & Golanty, 1992, p. 65). The American Diabetes Association (ADA) estimates that "3 million Black Americans have Diabetes . . . are 55% more likely to have diabetes, and 1 in every 10 Black Americans have Diabetes" (ADA, Diabetes Facts, 1990). Some literature suggests that diabetes was relatively uncommon during the beginning of this century. However, today it is the fourth leading cause of death among African-American women. Figure 1 presents the severity of this problem among African-American women.

As you can see from these comparative figures, the prevalence of diabetes among African-American women in 1983 was relatively high and, even though there has been some improvement, their disease rate is far greater when compared to that of nonminority males and females and minority males. Diabetes is having a devastating impact on the African-American

This chapter is dedicated to the memory of Nellie Arzelia Thornton, July 1945–November 1995, who loved children and served as the 14th National President of Jack & Jill of America, and was my friend.

Figure 1
Age Prevalence of Diabetes by Race, Sex, and Year in the United States, 1980–1990

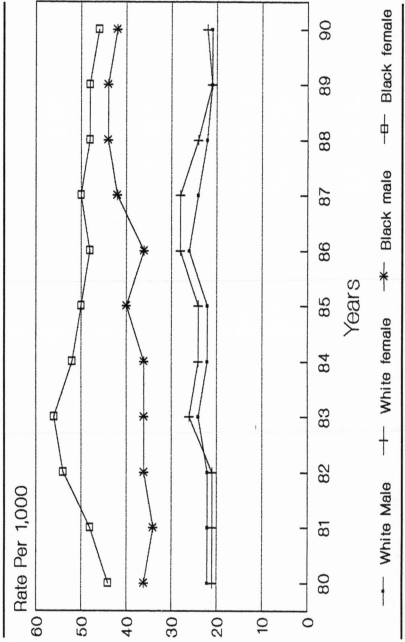

Rate Per 1,000

— White Male   + White female   * Black male   -□- Black female

Source: Adapted from *Diabetes Surveillance Report 1993*, p. 16.

community. In 1990 the National Institutes of Health reported that the number of African-American women diabetics can almost be termed an epidemic. The rate of diabetes in African-American women older than age 55 is one in four, double the rate of their white counterparts. As you can see in Figure 2, the rate of diabetes in African-American women increases significantly with age.

Diabetes is the end result of the body's inability to metabolize sugar and starch, which results in the accumulation of sugar in the blood. There are two types of diabetes; a brief description of both is offered. However, the impact of Type II non-insulin-dependent diabetes is the subject of this chapter. Briefly, Type I or insulin-dependent diabetes mellitus (IDDM), which requires daily injections of some form of insulin, usually has its onset during childhood years. Type II or non-insulin-dependent diabetes mellitus (NIDDM) is associated with the onset in the mature adult years. As you can see from Figure 2, the rate of diabetes in African-American women in their later years tops all others. Furthermore, Type II diabetes and its effects on the body, and the inability of the pancreas to produce enough insulin to regulate the amount of sugar in the individual's bloodstream, require the patient to control her diabetes by regulating her intake of food, through correct dietary management. One of the strong risk factors for acquiring Type II diabetes is obesity. With this in mind, diabetes requires careful management through continuous monitoring of lifestyle behavior and stress reduction management (SRM).

IMPACT OF THE HISTORICAL TREATMENT OF AFRICAN AMERICAN WOMEN AND THEIR HEALTH BEHAVIOR

In order to control lifestyle and inappropriate health behavior and practices, African-American women must have access to understandable health information from competent health care providers. African-American women who are knowledgeable about the historical mistreatment of their ancestors are often reluctant to trust the health system. Some have gained access to competent health care providers. However, "they are reminded that even with health access, their ancestors were subjected to discrimination and horrific medical abuses, such as injection with tuberculosis and syphilis bacteria, and impromptu limb amputation by white physicians eager to show medical students the latest surgical techniques" (Johnson, 1994, p. 54).

The media also help to further educate the American public regarding the atrocities committed by the medical profession. An example of this is the widely televised case of the African-American whose unaffected leg was mistakenly amputated by a Florida physician and in the traveling theater production of *Mrs. Evers' Boys*. This theater production of an accounting of an experiment called "The Tuskegee Study of Untreated Syphilis

Figure 2
Average Age Prevalence of Diabetes by Race, Sex, and Age in the United States, 1988–1990

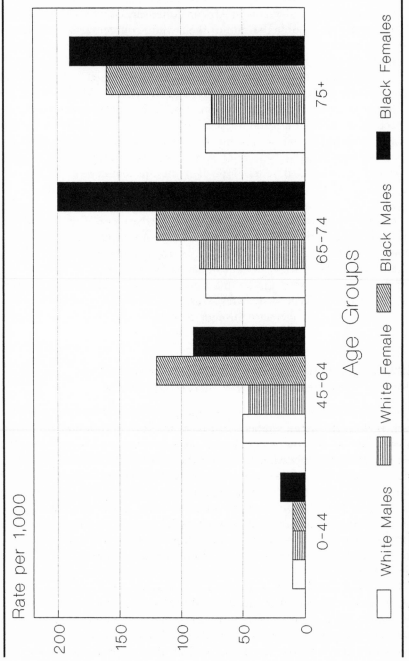

Rate per 1,000

Age Groups

White Males   White Female   Black Males   Black Females

Source: Adapted from Diabetes Surveillance Report 1993, p. 17.

in the Negro Male," authorized by the U.S. Public Health Service, sought to learn more about how syphilis actually attacks the body. The approach was to withhold treatment from 400 men, all poor, all black. These men were supervised by a public health nurse, Mrs. Evers. In the literature there are numerous historical accounts of the mistreatment of African-American women. Edward Beardsley's article, "Race as a Factor in Health" (1990), provided an excellent historical account of health care provided to African-American women. This historical account and others have helped create a sense of mistrust and apprehension among African-American women about seeking medical attention. In Beardsley's first historical account, "Era of Denial—1900–1930," he discusses how African-American women were denied access to health professionals and hospital services. This accounted for numerous childbirth deaths of both mothers and infants, as well as raging tuberculosis and syphilis. Also noted by Beardsley was the "scourge of American black women that also contributed to high morbidity—and death from other causes—diabetes mellitus. . . . Pre-1940 data are scanty, but current knowledge suggests that diabetes was a serious illness then, especially for women over 50" (p. 128).

MORTALITY AND RACISM IN THE AFRICAN-AMERICAN FEMALE ENVIRONMENT

There is, however, other evidence supported by government records, such as the *Report of the Secretary's Task Force on Black and Minority Health,* vol. VII: *Chemical Dependency and Diabetes* (1986). Statistics from surveys carried out in the early 1920s note the rise in the rates of non-insulin–dependent diabetes in blacks, particularly black women, as well as a higher rate of diabetes mortality and complications in the black community. As Beardsley (1990, p. 128) points out, cardiovascular and renal disease are severe complications of diabetes, and were, by 1900, among the greatest killers of blacks. African-American women, then (1900) and now (95 years later) still have the highest mortality according to U.S. government agencies. The *Diabetes Surveillance Report 1993* of the Division of Diabetes Translation at the Center for Disease Control and Prevention is a testament to the seriousness of the problem and the incredible death rate (see Table 7).

Furthermore, data from a second federal government document, *Health of the United States 1993,* show that African-American women's mortality rates, when compared to their white counterparts, are almost tripled (see Table 8).

As presented in Tables 7 and 8, the mortality rate from diabetes mellitus in African-American women is staggering. As Beardsley notes in the "Era of Inclusion 1930–1960," the access of African-American women to

Table 7
Number of Deaths with Diabetes as
Underlying Cause and Mortality Rates
per 100,000 Population by Age and
Year for Black Women in the United
States, 1980 and 1989

Age	1980	1989
45–54	26.00	25.00
55–64	69.40	81.50
65–74	146.50	162.20
75–84	221.90	279.80
85+	306.10	404.20

Source: Adapted from *Diabetes Surveillance
Report 1993,* Table 3-5, p. 38.

health services has increased because of the federal government's Hill Burton program, which provided resources to build hospitals. With federal
intervention, some hospitals admitted African-American women to segregated hospital wards. Many of these wards were understaffed, poorly
equipped, and attended by racist white physicians. The Great Depression
of this era also took its toll on African-Americans who were forced out of
jobs to make room for unemployed whites (Beardsley, 1990). Even though
African-American women were able to use hospital services in their communities, there were no guarantees that they would receive quality care.
Hospital policies impacted their care, where "expectant black mothers

Table 8
Age-Adjusted Diabetes Mortality Rates per 100,000
Residents, 1989, 1990, and 1991

	1989	1990	1991
Total Population	11.6	11.7	11.8
White Female	9.6	9.5	9.6
Black Female	24.6	25.4	25.7

Source: National Center for Health Statistics (1994), pp. 93–96.

were particularly victimized by Chicago racism: their own black hospitals often had no space for them, yet many maternity beds lay empty in white hospitals" (p. 137).

By the 1970s (Beardsley's "Era of Attempted Restitution") the Civil Rights Movement had opened some doors to health care. However, racism and its effects could still be found in hospitals built with federal dollars. In certain southern hospitals, African-American women could be hospitalized, but in segregated wards, often lacking equipment that was available in the white wards or wings of the same hospital. The Hill Burton federal program, coupled with other federal initiatives (Social Security), did not help with the incredible mortality rate of this era (see Table 8, 1989) where the death rate of black women was 60% above that of white and black men, with a rate of 45% (Beardsley, 1990, p. 138). Even with the programs previously mentioned, and the new programs of the 1990s, African-American women were still in poor health. From the data presented, it is evident that diabetes affects African-American women disproportionately. As such, there is no need for debate—it is a fact. What needs to be addressed is how we can impact on this plague.

All too often we look at socioeconomic status, poverty, access to health care, and level of education as the culprits in answering questions regarding the poor health status of African-American women. This is not to say that they are not contributors to ill health. However, when coupled with racism, the health status of African-American women is severely compromised. Racism, and the stress precipitated by it, is an etiologic factor in diabetes mellitus or diabetes complications, which must be considered in diseases that have such a deplorable outcome.

Racism and racists, who create stressful situations for African-American women, manipulate the environment in such a fashion that the stressor can affect the diabetic's physical well-being. Clearly, research has proven that stress will increase blood pressure (Newberry et al., 1991), heart rate (Edlin & Golanty, 1992), genital herpes recurrences (Schmidt, 1985), decreased renal excretion of salt resulting in increased fluid retention (Newberry et al., 1991), and yeast infection in college women (Williams and Deffenbacker, 1983). Furthermore, stress has been shown to impact on an individual's immune system, thus lowering resistance to infection, a complication of diabetes that often results in "black patients undergoing twice as many amputations as whites" (U.S. Dept. of Health, 1992).

There are many research studies which show that stress has an impact on the immune system. For example, dental students' antibody levels were significantly lowered before final examinations (Jemmott, 1984); and there is evidence that unemployed women had a reduction in white blood cells when compared to that of employed women (Armetz et al., 1987). Also, studies by Kiecolt-Glaser and Glaser in 1987 report of changes in immune systems of medical students during examinations and noted the impact of stress on recently separated women, when compared to married women's immune systems. There is no doubt that immunosuppression can be affected by stress. How severely the stress of racism will go in depressing the immune system function requires a much more in-depth approach, too lengthy for this chapter. However, as House (1986) puts it, "over a long run every stressful activity and subsequent adaptation wears us down biologically, contributing to aging, disease and eventual death." We must, therefore, control stressful situations arising out of racism. Is this possible?

According to a recently published article, "The Color of Health Care" (Johnson, 1994, p. 55) most African-Americans will be treated by white physicians [only 3% of U.S. physicians are black], "whose training and culture interfere with their good judgment. In short, their actions are racially motivated." Johnson continues to explain how racism rears its ugly head in the doctor's offices by presenting an analysis of a study by David Levy, a Houston family practitioner who investigated five ways race affects the doctor/patient relationship. As I present them, imagine that you are an overweight African-American female patient with diabetes mellitus.

According to Dr. Levy, racism raises its ugly head when a white physician shows his *disrespect* for a black patient by attending to a white patient who arrives after the black patient or begins the examination without introducing himself. On the other side is the white physician who *over-identifies* with a black patient, giving advice on how one should live one's life, or is *ignorant* of the importance of considering how African-American culture impacts on one's behavior. White physicians who proclaim to be color-blind in their care giving are also a detriment to the African-American patient, because these physicians fail to acknowledge the importance of race differences (e.g., health practices) that may need to be considered in the treatment plan. Dr. Levy's fifth example is the physician who makes assumptions about all African-Americans based on his experiences with a few. This physician *stereotypes* all African-Americans with the position where he believes they will all be without consideration of individual differences.

SOCIAL SUPPORT AND BUFFERS OF STRESS ASSOCIATED WITH RACISM AND DIABETIC PROGRAMS

African-American women who encounter the kind of racism described by Dr. Levy and other forms of racism (e.g., at work, at school) must shield themselves from the stress induced by these encounters. To buffer one's self from racism induced by our social and health care system, African-American women must turn to their social support network, which research has shown can mediate the impact of stressful life events and their effects on health outcomes.

Some have hypothesized that females with strong social support systems are much better prepared to cope with life stressors. Those who don't have strong social support systems can suffer dreadful results (e.g., poor physical and mental health). Social support can come from a variety of sources. One that appears to be key is the church, another is the family.

In research conducted by Brown and Gray (1987), entitled "Social Support and Physical and Mental Health of Urban Black Adults," 451 black adults (60% of whom were females) were studied to ascertain the level of relationship of social support and health outcomes. The following variables were used: nearby relatives, confidants, neighbors, religiosity, and perceived social support. One of the study's findings supports the importance of religious participation. It was noted "that increased frequency of participation in religious activities for black females is a way of coping with the ill health of loved ones and minimizing its effect on one's own physical health" (p. 171). Another study by Brown, Nilubuisi, and Gray (1990) noted that blacks with the least amount of religious participation had higher depressive symptoms, which further validates the importance of the church. However, there have been studies with mixed results, both positive and negative, regarding the effects of religion on depression (Dressler, 1991). When exploring the African-American church, women can and do "bring their problems to the Lord." This is done through the black church's rituals of "shouting," "dancing," deep religious meditation, testimonials, singing, and praising God. The theology of the sermon also serves as a teacher or counselor to help place the racist world into the context of the evil, mean-spirited antics of the devil. All of these rituals serve as tension relievers and as basic survival techniques. The congregations of black churches are disproportionately African-American females. No other institution has stood to aid the black community more than the black church. The church provides unlimited resources, food, shelter, counseling, and spiritual guidance (Wilmore, 1973). In the face of mounting social unrest of the 1960s, the church leadership (e.g., Dr. Martin Luther King) was the first social institution to publicly speak out against American racism. Thus the church provides a spiritual outlet for stress associated with racism.

The family also serves as an important social support network for African-American women. Historically, the absence of an American social structure that fosters social inclusion to help black women made them rely more heavily on what Staples (1991) termed the "mutual aid network," comprised of relatives, neighbors, and church members. This network provides much-needed services (e.g., baby-sitters). In Stock's (1974) study of poor inner-city black women, they found ways to devise mechanisms for sharing services, as well as means to cope with racism.

Obesity among African-American women is of epidemic proportions, and disproportionately so among black church congregations. Studies (Brown & Gray, 1987; Brown, Nilubuisi & Gray, 1990) show that religion and spirituality have some impact on the elevation of stress, which may affect diabetic outcomes. Such programs are now being instituted in church congregations. One such initiative—the Black Church Diabetic Program—was recently launched in the Los Angeles area. This program began with a kickoff breakfast for community leaders, to introduce them to the program's intent and concept. Health professionals from the American Diabetes Association and the chairman of the Cultural Diversity Program of the ADA were featured speakers, providing current evidence of the seriousness of diabetes among African-Americans nationwide. Utilizing the efforts of California Blue Cross, 200 churches were targeted for information sessions (Black Church Diabetes Program, 1994, p. A10). Information sessions allowed church participants to hear that diabetes is the third leading cause of death among African-Americans and gestational diabetes is recognized in 50% of pregnant black women.

Another similar program was initiated in my hometown of Buffalo, New York. The Cultural Diversity Program of the Western New York ADA spearheaded the church-congregation-directed program. A breakfast was also held with church pastors and other clergy to introduce them to the seriousness of diabetes among the community and their congregations. The diabetes program effort was appropriately entitled "Diabetes Sunday," and was presented to inner-city community block clubs and church congregations, who heard speakers and saw food demonstrations.

The black church is one of several avenues that can be used to reach at-risk overweight African-American women. Another is diabetes health education programs. One such program is PATHWAYS. Program participants were 13 NIDDM African-American women with a minimum of three months' treatment history and weighing at least 120% of ideal body weight (McNabb et al., 1993). The PATHWAYS program took reading levels into account to assure that the client could read educational materials, and utilized adult learning guidelines in presenting educational information. This program also gradually introduced dietary changes with a program guide that included ethnic foods (e.g., salt pork, ham hocks, greens) and a walking/exercise program. Of the 10 participants who completed the 18-week program, a loss of 9 to 10 pounds was noted, and after one year an average weight loss of 9.8 pounds was reported (McNabb et al., 1993). As the participants lost weight, their glycated hemoglobin values improved substantially. PATHWAYS included cultural considerations and adult learning style, which may have contributed significantly to its success. The program reported that behavior modification and lifestyle behavior changes were considered in working with this population. Religiosity as a variable was not mentioned in the PATHWAYS program design. However, because African-American women are in disproportionate numbers among the black church congregations, religiosity as a helping/reinforcement variable in health maintenance efforts (e.g., control weight gain) might be worth future investigation.

CONCLUSION

No one will deny that the health status of African-American women is poor, and a contributing factor is diabetes mellitus and its complications (e.g., blindness, amputation and end-stage renal disease) associated with poor health management and health practices. Epidemiological evidence clearly indicates that obesity, which is perpetuated by a "poverty diet" high in fats and sweets and low in vegetables and fruits, and a health care industry/social structure, which is riddled with racial discrimination and racism, both contribute to stress, lowering one's bodily defenses, and thus assuring poor health outcomes.

Furthermore, the impact on the health status of African-American women by those who are insensitive to cultural differences and the level of access they have to the health care industry/services will continue to increase health care cost with little or no return in healthy lifestyle. Heretofore, we have relied heavily on the health care industry to help alleviate the health ills of African-American women who suffer with diabetes. Efforts in diabetes health education have been designed to meet most of the physical health needs of African-American women. However, they need to be able to trust the system in order to feel comfortable in availing themselves of their services. These diabetic education programs have been designed most often within a medical or health behavioral model approach. Varying degrees of success have been noted in this chapter and in the literature. However, health educators must consider the impact of, and take a closer look at, how to utilize the spirituality of African-American women in program design. With the ever-increasing number of African-American women being diagnosed with NIDDM, both the traditional health education approach and the not so traditional (e.g., the church/spirituality) approach should be given serious consideration.

WORKS CITED

American Diabetes Association (1990). Diabetes facts (information fact sheet).

Armetz, B., Wasserman, B., Petreni, J. et al. (1987). Immune function in unemployed women, *Psychosomatic Medicine,* 49 (96), 3–12.

Beardsley, Edward (1990). Race as a factor in health. In Rima Apple, ed., *Women, Health and Medicine in America: A Historical Handbook.* New York: Garland.

Black church diabetes program gets underway in Los Angeles. (1994). Los Angeles *Sentinel,* September 22.

Brown, D. & Gray, L. (1987). Social support and physical and mental health of urban black adults. *Journal of Human Stress,* Winter, 165–174.

Brown, D., Nilubuisi, S., & Gray, L. (1990). Religiosity and psychological distress among blacks. *Journal of Religion and Health,* 29, 55–68.

Diabetes Surveillance Report 1993. (1993). Division of Diabetes Translation, Centers for Disease Control and Prevention, Atlanta.

Dressler, W. (1991). *Stress and Adaptation in the Context of Culture: Depression in a Southern Black Community.* Albany, NY: Albany University.

Edlin, G. & Golanty, E. (1992). *Health and Wellness: A Holistic Approach,* 4th ed. Boston: Jones and Bartlett.

Jemmott, J. B. III & Locke, S. E. (1984). Psychosocial factors, immunologic mediation, and human susceptibility to infectious diseases: How much do we know? *Psychological Bulletin,* 95, 78–108.

Johnson, K. A. (1994). The color of health care. *Heart and Soul,* Spring, 53–57.

Kiecolt-Glaser, J. K. & Glaser, R. (1987). Psychosocial moderators of immune functions. *Annals of Behavioral Medicine,* 9 (2), 16–20.

McNabb, W., Quinn, M. & Laurel, R. (1993). Weight loss program for inner-city black women with non-insulin dependent diabetes mellitus: PATHWAYS. *Journal of ADA,* 93, 75–77.

National Center for Health Statistics. (1994). *Health of the U.S. 1993.* Hyattsville, MD: Public Health Series, 93–96.

Newberry, B. H., Jaikin-Madden, J. & Gerstenberger, T. J. (1991). *A Holistic Conceptualization of Stress and Disease.* New York: Ams Press.

Report of the Secretary's Task Force on Black Minority Health. (1986). Vol. VII: *Chemical Dependency and Diabetes.* U.S. Department of Health and Human Services.

Schmidt, D. D., Zyanski, S., Ellner, J., Kumar, M. L., & Arno, J. (1985). Stress as a precipitating factor in recurrent herpes labialis. *Journal of Family Practice,* 20, 359–366.

Staples, R. (1991). *The Black Family Essays and Studies.* Belmont, CA: Wadsworth.

Stock, C. (1974). *All Our Kin: Strategies for Survival in a Black Community.* New York: Harper & Row.

U.S. Department of Health and Human Services. (1992). *Diabetes in Black Americans,* Fact Sheet. Washington, DC: NDIC Clearinghouse Publication, No. 93-326.

Wilmore, G. (1973). *Black Religion and Black Radicalism.* Garden City, NY: Anchor Books.

Williams, N. A. & Deffenbacker, J. L. (1983). Life stress and chronic yeast infections. *Journal of Human Stress,* 9, 26–31.

6

Alcohol Abuse and Stress Among African-American Women

Jacqueline D. Skillern Jackson

Straussner (1985), in her review of literature, found a history of references to alcohol abuse among African-American women covering an extensive span of time, if not in great quantity. She stated that Jellinek, as early as 1942, noted that the mortality rate of alcoholism among African-Americans was higher than whites and attributed the overall elevated rate among African-Americans to exceptionally high rates among African-American women. A 1965 New York City household survey showed a ratio of 1.9 to 1 African-American alcoholic males to females compared to 6.2 to 1 for white alcoholic males to females (Bailey et al., 1965). Cahalan and Cisin (1968), in a national random sample, found that while there were more African-American women who abstained from drinking (51%) compared to white women who abstained (39%), among those who did drink, there was a higher proportion of heavy drinkers (38%) as compared to white women (11%). Other studies done in the 1960s and 1970s continued to support the finding that there was a high prevalence of heavy drinking among African-American women (Caetano, 1984; Cahalan et al., 1974; and Bailey et al., 1965). Lillie-Blanton et al. (1991) found racial differences in their research examining characteristics of nondrinkers and heavy drinkers in Baltimore. They found that African-American women between the ages of 18 and 24, or older than 60, or who were married were more likely to be nondrinkers than white women in those categories. They further discovered that women of both groups with 12 years or more of formal education were less likely to be heavy drinkers. Among heavy drinkers, African-American women peaked between the ages of 45 and 59 and for white women the peak was between 25 and 44. There was a high correlation of alcohol abuse or dependence among both black and white women between 25 and 50 (particularly 45–59 for black women) with annual incomes of less than $6,000 and who were separated, divorced, or widowed.

In attempting to understand the overrepresentation of African-American women in the heavy drinking/alcoholic population, it would be helpful to examine some of the etiological factors contributing to alcohol abuse among women. Beckman (1976) stated that women tend to show escapist drinking and that alcoholism and heavy drinking among women appeared to be linked to psychological stress and specific precipitating circumstances. Straussner (1985) came to a similar conclusion, stating that for poor women alcoholism was socially induced, while for middle-class women it was more closely related to psychological factors. She went on to say that African-American women show high patterns of both abstinence and alcoholism. She further indicated that poor women who drink have a higher rate of alcoholism.

STRESS AND ADDICTION

There has been a general consensus among researchers that the etiological factors of psychological stress, precipitating circumstances or situations, and lower socioeconomic status are major contributing factors to alcohol abuse among women in general and African-American women specifically. This chapter presents a theoretical framework that examines contributing factors to alcohol abuse among African-American women and more closely looks at some of the specific psychological stressors and circumstances that place African-American women at risk for high levels of alcohol abuse and alcoholism.

Stress is the physiological, psychological, and emotional response to changes in one's internal and external environment (Adams, 1980). A certain amount of stress is necessary to live and for the most part is harmless (Sharpe & Lewis, 1977). Healthy stress occurs when there is a balance between clear, realistic demands and adequate resources available to meet those demands. In ordinary situations, when individuals experience stress, they access internal or external resources to meet the demands or attempt to adjust the demands to maintain homeostasis. When there is an imbalance between the demands and the resources at one's disposal to meet those demands, one experiences unhealthy stress. Unhealthy stress over a period of time leads to distress. Distress, again over time, results in the deterioration of one's ability to develop and access resources or to manage demands. Eventually, with prolonged distress, one's focus shifts from resource development and demand management toward pain relief. When seeking relief, the quest is for an agent that is quick, easy, effective, and available (cost and proximity). Unfortunately, agents meeting those qualifications often have the additional quality of being self-destructive. Thus the stress/distress model of addiction is as follows: an imbalance between demands and resources to meet those demands → distress; distress + time → a reduced ability to access healthy relief → focus shift away from resource development and demand management to pain relief→ self-destructive behaviors (alcohol abuse)→ downward spiral into addiction (alcoholism).

Demands placed on African-American women include external demands (those placed by others) and internal demands (those placed by oneself). The internal demands often represent internalized external demands. Whether internal or external, the demands become problematic stressors when they are unrealistic, unclear, and/or inappropriate. For African-American women, the stressors often take the form of distorted role expectations about them as African-Americans and as women. They are constantly judged by others in their families and communities against standards and norms based on myths, stereotypes, and unhealthy expectations. Stressors for African-American women can be categorized as historical/generational, internal, and external (environmental) (the latter will be discussed in a later section of this chapter).

Historical/Generational Stressors

Historical/generational stressors are those events that have historically or perpetually had a negative impact on the self-esteem of African-American women. These events have directly or indirectly invalidated their needs and their right to have those needs addressed. Probably the oldest and most significant historical event was slavery (being sold, raped, and bred at the will of others). The message that was given to African-American women and to the world about African-American women was that they were a commodity, less than human. They were considered inferior to men, with no rights or privileges. They were both politically and economically powerless. After slavery, African-American women remained in the same low status. They were expected to be satisfied with being producers and caretakers (having children, raising both their own and the children of others, and caring for the physical and psychological needs of their families as well as the families for whom they worked, most often as domestic servants). Personal needs were neither recognized nor validated, and there were no mechanisms to address those needs. African-American women have been and continue to be expected to function as superwomen

in the presence of the message that they are politically, economically, physically, and psychologically inferior. The dissonance created by attempts to
fulfill astronomical behavioral expectations while, at the same time, being
treated as inconsequential and inferior has and continues to place African-
American women at high risk for alcohol abuse and alcoholism.

Internal Stressors

Internal stressors that place African-American women at high risk for
alcohol abuse and alcoholism are those issues that are generated within
the individual or the internalization of ideas, concepts, and constructs generated by others that affect behavior. Two primary groups of such issues
are the myths and stereotypes about African-American women and four
major areas of individual functioning that singularly and collectively determine internal stress levels, which in turn increase or decrease the risk of
alcohol abuse and alcoholism.

MYTHS AND STEREOTYPES ABOUT
AFRICAN-AMERICAN WOMEN

The rational-emotive approach to behavior developed by Albert Ellis
states that emotional or behavioral consequences are not determined by
activating events (antecedents), but by one's cognitive mediations, as fil-
tered through one's belief system about those events. This includes one's
perceptions, inferences, and conclusions (Ellis, 1977). The theory further
postulates that, to the extent that cognitive mediations (belief systems) are
realistic, rational, and oriented toward the optimal functioning of the individual, consequent behavior will be adaptive and appropriate for growth,
development, and health. If, however, the cognitive mediations are faulty,
irrational, or serve to perpetuate invalid constructs, resultant behavior will
be dysfunctional. Thus, to understand, change, or prevent dysfunctional
behavior, one must examine cognitive mediations and the constructs on
which they are based to determine their validity and appropriateness for a
given issue, event, or situation.

Applying a rational emotive approach to understanding African-American women as a high-risk population for alcohol abuse and alcoholism is
not just the result of the antecedent being African-American and female,
as there are indeed African-American women who do not abuse alcohol.
Rather, it is the faulty cognitive mediations of some African-American
women about being African-American and female that results in dysfunctional, high-risk behavior. To the extent that one's cognitions, perceptions,
inferences, and conclusions about being African-American and female are
realistic, valid, and oriented toward optimal personal functioning, resultant behaviors will reflect a low alcohol abuse risk factor. Conversely, cog-

nitive mediations that are faulty and/or serve to perpetuate invalid constructs increase the risk aspect of alcohol abuse and alcoholism. For African-American women who abuse alcohol, the latter is often the case. Their cognitive mediations often reflect the internalization of invalid assumptions, standards, and norms that, for the most part, have been externally generated.

Internalization of myths and stereotypes about African-American women that have been perpetuated over time represent some of the most hazardous cognitive mediations. The majority of these myths and stereotypes represent conflictive and dysfunctional standards of behavior that retard, if not prohibit, personal growth and development. Conscious or subconscious attempts of African-American women to act in accordance with these myths and stereotypes produce stress and dissonance, thus increasing the risk of dysfunctional behavior—in this case alcohol abuse and alcoholism. Listed below are some of the most commonly held myths and stereotypes about African-American women collected from workshop participants conducted by this author during the past seven years.

African-American Women

1. are competent only in the kitchen and bedroom
2. are unclear about the real meaning of life by virtue of being African-American
3. are domineering
4. are always ventilating
5. are castrating
6. are superwomen
7. are competitive
8. are distrustful
9. are disrespectful
10. are all alike
11. are unable to hold positions of responsibility
12. are paranoid
13. are too independent
14. are hard headed, cannot teach them anything
15. are victims
16. are too possessive
17. do not appreciate good treatment; must be shown who is boss
18. are the salt of the earth
19. are always angry or hostile
20. are more cunning than African-American males
21. are not hurt by anything

22. want to be men

23. are more emotional than African-American males

24. dress nice

25. are unable to figure out; one can never tell where they are coming from

26. are sexy

27. have too many problems for *anything* to do any good

28. are too vocal

29. are fat

30. are suffering

31. cannot get along with each other

32. are not supportive of African-American men

33. only get along well with each other

34. are matriarchal

35. are uneducated

36. are church goers

37. have a lot of children

38. are materialistic

39. are on welfare

40. are isolated

41. are wise

42. are happy

43. are erotic

44. like each other

45. are strong and do not need to ask for help

46. are hysterical

47. enjoy taking care of others

48. do not know their place

49. have to be right

50. are forgiving

51. are more in touch with their feelings than African-American males

52. are loud

It is important to note that many of the stereotypes conflict with each other. Examples of such conflicts include: "are superwomen"—"are victims," "cannot get along with each other"—"only get along well with each other," "are always angry or hostile"—"are happy," "are unable to hold positions of responsibility"—"are strong and do not need to ask for help," "are castrating"—"are forgiving," "are hysterical"—"are more in touch with their feelings than African-American males." These contradictions leave the black woman's behaviors often judged and responded to as simultaneously appropriate and inappropriate. Stress comes from functioning in an environment in which one is judged as right and wrong at the same time, and given mixed messages about appropriate and inappropriate behavior.

INDIVIDUAL LEVELS OF FUNCTIONING

Research conducted at Fanon Research Center (King, 1982) identified four primary areas that determine the optimal functioning of an individual: physical-biological, political-economic, psychosocial, and spiritual. Depending on how well each of these areas is functioning individually and collectively, the individual experiences more or less stress. The greater the stress, the higher the risk for alcohol abuse. In examining these areas as they relate to African-American women, we find that in all four areas African-American women have historically experienced and continue to experience disharmony.

Physical-Biological Functioning

The physical-biological area of functioning includes basic needs such as food, shelter, and health care. For many African-American women, stress in this area reflects the substandard living conditions that accompany forced poverty and discrimination (racial and sexual). External environmental stressors to which African-American women are exposed include crowding, excessive air and noise pollution, inadequate housing, violence, crime, drug-related crime including homicide, and higher housing costs leading to an inflated cost of living (Edwards et al., 1994a; Laveist, 1993).

African-American women are overrepresented as female heads of household as well as among the poor. As of 1990, 43.8% of African-American families were female head of household with a median family income of $12,125; 29.3% of families were at poverty and 31.9% were below poverty as defined by the U.S. Office of Management and Budget (Edwards et al., 1994a). Amaro et al., (1987) compared African-American women and white women in alcohol treatment facilities and found that 50% of the African-American women in the study were separated and more than 25% had never married, compared to the white women, of whom 38% were divorced, 19% separated, and 10% never married. Consistent with poverty and single head-of-household status is the lack of adequate affordable housing, substandard clothing, poor nutrition, in many instances the lack of transportation, and poor health due to inadequate health care.

In looking at health issues for African-American women, we see that there are internal biological stressors such as high rates of hypertension, lactose intolerance, and obesity that contribute to their high-risk health status. Highlighted as an external biological stressor for African-American women is the issue of health care. We see that many African-American women either are unable to afford adequate health care on their own, are in jobs that do not have adequate health care plans, or are ineligible to use the plans because they have not worked at the job long enough to qualify for health care benefits. To this group add those who are unable to use the health care plans of significant others or the fathers of their children because they are not married. Amaro et al. (1987) found that 10 times as many white women as African-American women in alcohol treatment had health insurance coverage.

Studies show that even when health care is available, African-American women access it at lower rates than white women. Researchers hypothesized that perhaps blacks were unable to take advantage of availability for reasons such as transportation problems, child-care arrangements, inflexible employment schedules, lower levels of satisfaction with their care and other factors, and the cultural perceptions of the value of preventive health care.

Another major physical-biological stressor for African-American women is the high infant mortality and morbidity of African-American infants. African-American women are twice as likely as women from other ethnic groups to have babies with low birth weights and to experience the loss of infant death (Hogue & Hargraves, 1993; Gates-Williams et al., 1992; Mitchell, 1990). The infant mortality rate for whites in 1993 ranked 12th compared to other industrialized countries, while the rate for blacks was 26th, bordering on the rates for Third World developing nations (Laveist, 1993).

Thus, in the physical-biological area, we see many African-American women experiencing stress in the most basic areas of functioning, which in turn places them at high risk for alcohol abuse.

Political-Economic Functioning

The political-economic area focuses on one's relationship to and position in political and economic arenas. This includes educational status, occupational status, employment, income, earnings, and the amount of control and power individuals have over themselves and their environment.

Major political stressors discussed in the literature for African-American women are racism, the impact of bureaucracy on one's life, and the impact of segregation. Economic stressors include unemployment, underemployment, lack of educational and career opportunities, as well as the problems most commonly associated with poverty and inner-city lifestyles.

Racism. While most would not like to acknowledge it, racism has been part of the fabric of America since its beginning. Each new wave of immigrants has been the victim of prejudice and discrimination by those who were already here. While some European cultures who immigrated to this country over time were able to assimilate, the salience of color has left others in a situation of continuing experiences of prejudice, discrimination, and racism simply because of their membership in a certain race or ethnic group. In spite of the Civil Rights laws, desegregation, equal opportunity, affirmative action, and the present-day focus on diversity, racism has continued not only to have a presence but to negatively impact the lives of those who experience its consequences. While not as blatant and overt as in the past, with beating, lynchings, and enslavement, modern racism in the form of redlining, police brutality, discrimination in job hiring and promotion practices, and overrepresentation of people of color in the criminal justice arena all are stressors that serve as barriers to healthy lifestyles for African-Americans (Edwards et al., 1994a). One of the many consequences of being a victim of racism is the loss of self-esteem and the intensification of the feeling of helplessness.

Bureaucracy. With increasing technology, bureaucracy management has become more stressful. As the size and scope of agencies have increased, their supporting infrastructures have become more complex, cumbersome, rigid, and, thus, less user friendly. Many of the stressors originating from interactions with bureaucracies can be characterized into those issues that serve as barriers to access and those associated with services received. Russell and Jewell (1992) detail four primary barriers to service experienced by African-American pregnant women: their inability to pay for services, lack of transportation and child care, decreased understanding of health-related treatment plans, and difficulty incorporating prescribed treatment plans into their daily living. Other authors highlighted stressors associated with the quality of health care received. Literature shows that African-American patients tend to receive less intensive hospital services and are less likely to be satisfied with the care they receive from physicians and hospitals. They are not served well by city services and receive low-quality social and public services. They also reported difficulties with transportation, child care arrangements, and inflexible employment schedules when trying to access services (Edwards et al., 1994a, Pursley & Wise, 1992, Laveist, 1993, Murray & Bernfield, 1988).

Economic Stressors. Economic stressors experienced by African-American women place them at risk. Not only have they been in a historical position of powerlessness in society, often associated with being poor, but according to the U.S. Bureau of the Census (1987), they experience high levels of unemployment and underemployment (45% unemployment rate among poor African-American women); lack of career opportunities (as of 1981 only 30% of African-American women had positions in the workforce as professionals or clerical help), and inadequate education (as of 1985 only 11% of African-American women had completed college). This is placed against a background of the constant experience of sexism (being subjugated to a rigidly defined place and role in society) and racism (being relegated to second-class citizenship).

Several authors refer to the economic and demographic stressors associated with being African-American, living in the inner cities, and being poor. They indicated that African-Americans in inner cities have greater exposure to environmental pollution, have higher crime and incarceration rates, spend fewer years in school, have higher levels of unemployment and underemployment, have less income and wealth resulting in greater numbers of black women and children in poverty, live in more dilapidated housing, have a higher incidence of teen pregnancy, experience a lack of adequate medical care, and are exposed to a lower quality of social and public services (Edwards et al., 1994a, 1994b; Russell & Jewell, 1992; Editorial, 1992, Gould, Davey & LeRoy, 1989).

Psychosocial Functioning

The psychosocial area includes relationships, interpersonal interactions, and participation in social and institutional support systems. For African-American women, psychosocial stressors include, as previously discussed, dissonance created by behavior that reflects internalized myths and stereotypes about being African-American and female, low self-esteem, peer pressure, the depression and hopelessness that often accompany poverty, the lack of socialization of African-American women into supportive communities and families, issues of sexuality, relationship issues (mother-child, female-female, and female-male), and the lack of knowledge about developing, accessing, and participating in support systems.

For many African-American women, a major stressor is the extreme isolation and loneliness experienced as the result of living in an inner-city, overcrowded situation (Smith & Draper, 1994). While surrounded by many others in similar conditions, these women often feel that interacting with or developing relationships with those beyond one's immediate family increases the risk of added "confusion," stress, and the general fear for safety. Isolation and loneliness are often compounded by the absence of support from a male partner. For some women, a stable relationship with a male partner is someone with whom to share, a stress mitigator, and, in some instances, represents physical safety. At the same time, social support by family or significant others becomes a cognitive mediator against the environment. The absence of a healthy support system leaves a woman isolated and lonely, negatively impacting her anxiety and self-esteem. High anxiety was found to be associated with low self-esteem, a high number of disagreements with partners, a low amount of time spent with partners, a lower degree of happiness in relationships with partners, and, thus, a smaller social network (Edwards et al., 1994a; Smith & Draper, 1994).

High stress levels can cause self-isolation, resulting in reduced contacts with people and relationships that could serve as mediators to their stress, or lead to being so overwhelmed that one is unable to effectively access and use the relationships that are available. This, in turn, may result in depression and learned helplessness as well as detrimental physiological and psychological symptoms. Research found that the smaller the social network, the greater one's anxiety about oneself (Edwards et al., 1994a).

A further stressor for African-American women is the double standard that exists regarding women and alcohol consumption and the impact of that double standard on how women who drink are perceived. Lisansky-Gomberg and Nirenberg (1991), in summarizing the literature, found that there are far more women who drink moderately and within socially acceptable limits than there are excessive drinkers. However, they found that norms, values, attitudes, and expectations are different for women than for men. While most societies permit women to drink in moderation, there is more of a negative view of female intoxication than male intoxication. They summarized earlier research by Knupfer in 1964, which stated that female intoxication was considered an impairment to nurturant behavior and intoxicated women were viewed as more sexually available and, thus, often considered morally loose. The stressor for African-American women, then, is that they are expected to participate in a socially acceptable behavior within the black community (drinking), but are also expected to do so within a narrower set of boundaries than men. If the boundaries are crossed, the social price is much greater for women than for men.

Spiritual Functioning

Spirituality issues include values, beliefs, customs, lifestyles, religion, and the extent to which and manner in which they are expressed. While this area has historically contained some of the primary stressors for African-American women such as double standards, myths, and strong sexism, it has also been an area from which African-American women have experienced tremendous support. Russell and Jewell (1992), in reviewing studies conducted by Spector in 1985 on the historical role of religion and health, found that African-Americans viewed health on a continuum, and saw the mind, body, and spirit as linked. When ill, God was seen as a healer, accessed through prayer. Illness was alleviated by God's will and one's faith in God. Health was seen as a blessing from God and God was seen as protecting individuals. By being close to God, one was protected from harm and when illness occurred, a common response was to pray for God's protection and cure. Thus, for African-American people in general, and African-American women specifically, spirituality has existed as a source of strength, identity, and empowerment. It has been seen as a means of protection, enrichment, and expansion. Whether structured or unstructured, spirituality has historically been the primary mediator of both internal and external stressors for African-American women.

In each major area of functioning that has been discussed, African-American women are experiencing stressors that individually and collectively elevate their overall stress levels. These increased stress levels, often in the absence of effective mediators and resources, place them at high risk for alcohol abuse and alcoholism.

EXTERNAL (ENVIRONMENTAL) STRESSORS

While many issues that negatively affect African-American women originate from within, other issues are externally generated (environmental stressors), primarily from the family and the community.

Family Stressors

Researchers have written about African-American families since the 1960s. They have identified family structures and dynamics that have facilitated the survival of the black family through tumultuous and stressful times. Stevenson and Renard (1993) summarized the works of Billingsley, Hill, Christophenson, Royce and Turner, and Boykin and Toms to provide a historical perspective of the strengths of African-American families written between 1968 and 1985. Some of those characteristics, while good for the family as a whole, have been costly for African-American women, often requiring the sacrifice of their individual growth, development, and optimal functioning. Several of the family characteristics that have placed women's individuality under stress are the African-American family organizational structure, women's role regarding the strong kinship bonds in the family, a strong achievement orientation in the family, and the family approach to the expression of feelings.

Organization. Family organization in the African-American family is well ordered regarding family activities and plans. Rules and responsibilities are clear and concise (Wynne, 1985). While roles may be flexible or interchangeable among family members, the responsibilities or behaviors that accompany those roles are rigid. For African-American women, this can be stressful because they are often required to assume several roles simultaneously, each geared toward family survival with behavioral codes that do not allow for individual needs to exist or to be met. As has been the case historically, they continue in the role of physical and psychological caretaker of others.

Kinship Bonds. The African-American family has strong kinship bonds. There is an overriding concern for family unity, for loyalty to the family unit, and an emphasis on cooperation rather than competition among family members (Wynne, 1985). For African-American women this not only continues to perpetuate their role as caretaker of others, but serves as a barrier to women expressing their needs and getting those needs met within the family. Since loyalty to, service to, and perpetuation of the family as a unit is the primary focus, anything that emphasizes or brings attention to any measure smaller than the family is considered invalid and is looked upon with disfavor. Acknowledging and attending to individual needs and concerns are seen as disloyal and disruptive to the unit, as fostering competition within the unit, and, as a consequence, are discouraged. In response to African-American women who act in self-destructive ways when their individual needs are unmet, we hear phrases like "how could she do that to her family," "her children don't deserve that," "going against her family like that."

Achievement. Within African-American families, achievement is highly valued (Wynne, 1985). Family members are encouraged to be competitive outside the family and the extent of one's achievements often determines value. For African-American women, this ethic can be stressful, because the avenues available to behave in ways consistent with the value are often limited. The reality is that African-American women continue to be one of the most disenfranchised groups in our society today. For the most part they are underemployed, underpaid, undereducated, and politically and economically powerless. In other words, African-American women have few real opportunities to compete in our society, and, thus, have fewer "tangible achievements" to show, which in turn diminishes them as not exemplifying valued behavior within the family.

Expression. Within the African-American family, for the most part, family members are encouraged to express their thoughts and feelings (Wynne, 1985). Verbal skills of African-Americans and the ability to "speak one's mind," to "tell it like it is," have long been recognized among African-American people. The ability to speak up for oneself is encouraged. African-American women, however, are in a double-bind in this area. As caretakers, their roles have been to care for the emotional and psychological needs of others first and their own second, if at all. Thus, the things women say, the feelings they express, must be tempered so as to be facilitative of the well-being of others. Expressing their needs, which may or may not be in concert with the needs of others, is dampened in order to maintain the caretaker/facilitator role. A second point of stress in this area is the stereotype about verbal expression and African-American women. One of these myths or stereotypes is that they are too sharp-tongued. Aware of this stereotype, African-American women must verbally conduct themselves in concert with the value of verbal expression, but be mindful of the stereotype. Consequently, they are in a bind. If they express themselves and their needs too much, they are being sharp-tongued and may be seen as emotionally or psychologically damaging to other family members. On the other hand, if they don't express themselves enough, they are not living up to family values.

For the most part, the family issues that place black women under stress, and thereby increasing their risk of alcohol abuse, are those issues that require them to function primarily for the development and enhancement of the family unit without mechanisms for the recognition and resolution of their individual needs.

Community Stressors

The community contributes stressors to African-American women by continuing to view them in stereotypical ways and by placing upon them the unrealistic expectation of behaving in accordance with norms and guidelines that the community has developed and that seldom reflect women's individual needs. For the most part, the norms and guidelines are conflictual and trivialize, if not entirely deny, the existence of African-American women's personal growth and development needs. Consequently, the community provides neither mechanisms nor a supportive environment in which their needs can be addressed. At the community level, African-American women either attempt to live the community agenda, which causes personal dissonance, or experience the ostracism and criticism when they don't live up to community-generated expectations that are often based on myths and stereotypes. To choose the latter increases the risk of being labeled as uncaring, unfeeling, not a good wife, mother, lover, and so on. In both cases black women would experience the hopelessness of trying to get individual needs met in an environment void of the resources to do so. They experience stress and frustration, which place them at high risk for a focus shift toward pain relief—usually in the form of self-destructive behavior.

Caetano (1984) found that attitudes toward drinking are more liberal among African-American women and men than among white women and men. However, fewer African-American women than white women approve of women "getting drunk." Amaro et al. (1987) interpreted Caetano's results to mean that while African-American women may live in social environments with more liberal norms with respect to drinking, there is not necessarily a more liberal norm regarding female intoxication. This thinking is evident in the intensity of negative community response to and absence of support available for African-American women when they have drinking problems.

Belle (1982) found that while some poor single African-American mothers had more contact with a social network than their white counterparts, they often experienced more demands and stress than support from those networks. In looking at the social fabric of these women's lives, it is important to realize that contact does not necessarily equal support. In fact, the internalization of the caretaker role to the exclusion of self and the lack of perceived personal support can result in feelings of aloneness, alienation, and isolation consistent with the results found by Amaro et al. (1987). The increase in demands with increased contact further supports the historical/generational role of African-American women as caretakers of the physical, emotional, and psychological needs of others with little focus and/or ability to address their own needs.

Thus, in the community, with an external focus on taking care of others, coupled with a denial of self, African-American women may find themselves surrounded by the needs of others to which they feel compelled to respond, yet significantly stressed due to their own personal needs. Consistent with a stress/distress model, their focus can quickly shift from resource development to pain relief, thus increasing the risk of alcohol abuse and addiction.

PREVENTION STRATEGIES FOR ALCOHOL ABUSE AND ALCOHOLISM

For African-American women to avoid the pitfalls of alcohol abuse and alcoholism, the addiction formula must be addressed. As stated earlier, distress occurs when there is an imbalance between demands and resources. We have discussed the demands, the absence of resources, and how the interplay between those two factors places African-American women at risk. To balance the equation, resource identification and access must be a priority. Resources are the people, places, and things that assist in handling the internal and external demands. Just as demands came from both internal and external sources, so do resources.

Internal Resources

The development of internal resources includes developing and accessing people, places, and things to assist one in challenging demands, and/or developing resources consistent with those demands. Internal resources include self-empowerment, stress recognition, knowledge of agencies, individual knowledge about alcohol and consequences of alcohol abuse, and an increased ability to critically examine both internal and external demands.

Recognition. A primary resource need is the ability to recognize the symptoms of stress within oneself. Too often women do not recognize that they are experiencing unhealthy stress until it is too late. And even then, stress activates the cognition that "I am not doing something right and must do more." Women must be taught to recognize when the imbalance between resources and demands is occurring before they reach the stage of focus shift to pain relief. African-American women must learn to recognize the physical, emotional, psychological, and environmental stressors that place them at risk. Along with recognition of an imbalance in the equation, African-American women must recognize the self-statements that reflect their distress and see those as signals of prefocus shift behavior. They must learn to recognize not only when they are experiencing stress, but learn the cues that indicate they may be expressing distress.

Self-Empowerment. Self-empowerment includes moving women from hoping it will get better to making it better for themselves. African-American women must be taught and encouraged to successfully and adequately address their political, economic, and spiritual needs. They must broaden the arena of "who they care for" to include themselves without apology and become unwilling to forego getting their own needs met in favor of others.

Critical Thinking. African-American women must learn to critically examine both the internal and external demands placed upon them for reality and appropriateness. Rather than internalize distorted community expectations and norms, African-American women must learn to determine for themselves appropriate behavioral responses to stimuli in their environment. Critical thinking involves understanding, assessment, and response. African-American women must understand the demands made on them, assess the reality and appropriateness of those demands, and determine an effective response to those demands based on healthy models of behaving rather than a model of self-sacrifice at all costs. African-American women must learn to challenge the myths about them, and learn to prevent and interrupt the internalization of those myths, which often lead to the consequent self-destructive behavior of alcohol abuse.

Resource Development. African-American women must become aware of and more knowledgeable about the agencies, institutions, and relationships that can adequately address their needs, and learn how to access those systems for assistance. Too often the paperwork and procedures for assistance amount to locked doors for African-American women. Already feeling guilty, embarrassed, selfish, and ashamed for needing and seeking help for themselves, African-American women are easily deterred by bureaucratic procedures that seem to reinforce the inappropriateness of seeking help.

Self-Advocacy Skills. In addition to learning which agencies, institutions, programs, and relationships are available to address their needs, African-American women must learn to access those services. Furthermore, they must learn to participate in the adjustment of those services to better meet their needs rather than withdrawing from participation because programs are insensitive. They must become their own most powerful advocates and help others to become true resources rather than demands masquerading as resources.

Increased Awareness. African-American women must be educated about the negative consequences of alcohol abuse and addiction. They must learn of the physical, psychological, and emotional problems directly and indirectly associated with alcohol abuse and addiction.

External Resources

External resources primarily include community strategies to recognize and address those issues that place African-American women at high risk for distress and subsequent alcoholism. These strategies may include environmentally based issues such as employment, health care, education, vocational training, and child care, but they will also address alcohol-specific issues such as cultural attitudes and mores toward alcohol use and abuse, the establishment of norms and guidelines about alcohol consumption, and the institution of public policies and laws governing the use and availability of alcohol in the community. The community must become adept not only at recognizing those issues that negatively impact African-American women but at identifying and mobilizing resources to address those concerns. The community can insure adequate resources by focusing on validation, sensitivity, community education, and community development.

Validation. Communities must develop mechanisms for validating the needs of African-American women and protect each woman's right to have those needs met in healthy ways. The community must, as African-American women must, become adept at recognizing issues that place African-American women at high risk and, further, fully understand the magnitude of the risk.

Sensitivity. Agencies and institutions serving women must become sensitive to the needs of women of color. It must be recognized that women are not shadows of men, that while they have similarities in some areas, they also have significantly different needs in other areas. Agencies must be sensitive to the enormity of the step of seeking help. Many tend to underestimate what African-American women have already accomplished before they come in the door. They have already violated community "norms," decided to risk community "punishment" not only for having the problem, but for going "public." Yet agencies, institutions, and people treat them as if they have just begun the journey to recovery and that they must start it with paperwork.

Community Development. The community must establish an environment that is supportive of African-American women rather than punitive. The message must be one of recognizing, celebrating, and protecting the rights of African-American women. With this comes valuing and nurturing African-American women rather than measuring their worth by their level of service to others.

Guidelines and Norms. The community must support the development of practices, norms, and guidelines about alcohol use that are gender-specific. Currently, women often determine their behavior patterns by copying, mimicking, or shadowing the behavior of men, assuming that male drinking styles are appropriate and that shadowing their behavior will meet their needs.

External resources must include family, community, and agency approaches to the issues of African-American women. The community must position itself to make realistic, appropriate demands on African-American women and to provide resources for African-American women to respond to demands in healthy ways. Alcohol abuse must be targeted as an unhealthy response to stress and viewed as a mechanism that will exacerbate rather than alleviate whatever stress African-American women may be experiencing.

CONCLUSION

In the stress-distress model of alcohol abuse, African-American women experience greater demands (internal and external) and fewer resources (internal and external) than their white counterparts. The magnitude of the equation imbalance between demands and resources places them at greater risk for self-destructive behavior—in this case, alcoholism. To bring this equation into balance, or to at least make it more manageable for African-American women, strategies must be developed that approach the equation from individual, community, and institutional approaches. African-American women must be strengthened to individually challenge the demands placed on them, and remain in a resource development mode to address those demands rather than shifting to a pain-relief mode. Communities must also examine how they contribute to the equation imbalance by making unreasonable demands and providing inadequate resources to meet those demands. Agencies and institutions must insure that their services are truly resources and do not add to the demand side of the equation. Thus, African-American women themselves, their community, and service agencies must all work to insure that the demands and resources for African-American women remain balanced, thereby reducing the risk of self-destructive behavior in the form of alcohol abuse and alcoholism.

WORKS CITED

Adams, J. D. (Ed.) (1980). *Understanding and Managing Stress: A Book of Readings.* San Diego: University Associates.
Amaro, H., Beckman, L. J. & Mays, V. M. (1987). A comparison of black and

white women entering alcoholism treatment. *Journal of Studies on Alcohol,* 43 (3), 220–228.

Bailey, M. B., Haberman, P. W. & Alksne, H. (1965). The epidemiology of alcoholism in an urban residential area. *Quarterly Journal on the Study of Alcohol,* 26, 19–40.

Beckman, L. J. (1976). Alcoholism problems and women: An overview. In M. Greenblatt & M. A. Schuckit, eds., *Alcoholism Problems in Women and Children.* New York: Grune & Stratton.

Belle, D. (ed.). (1982). *Lives in Stress: Women and Depression.* Beverly Hills, CA: Sage Publications.

Caetano. R. (1984). Ethnicity and drinking in northern California: A comparison among whites, blacks, and hispanics. *Alcohol and Alcoholism,* 19, 31–44.

Cahalan, D. & Cisin, I. (1968). American drinking practices: Summary of findings from a national probability sample. *Journal of Studies on Alcohol,* 29, 130–151.

Cahalan, D., Roizen, R. & Room, R. (1974). Alcohol problems and their prevention: Public attitudes in California. In R. Room & S. Sheffield, eds., *The Prevention of Alcohol Problems.* Report of a Conference. Sacramento: Office of Alcoholism, Health and Welfare Agency, 354–403.

Edwards, C. H., Cole, O. J., Oyemade, U. J. & Knight E. M. (1994a). Maternal Stress and Pregnancy Outcomes in a Prenatal clinic population. *Journal of Nutrition,* 124 (6 Supp), 1006S–1021S.

Edwards, C. H., Knight, E. M. & Johnson, A. A. (1994b). Multiple factors as mediators of reduced incidence of low birth rate in an urban clinic population. *Journal of Nutrition,* 124 (6 Supp), 927S–935S.

Ellis, A. & Grieger, R. (1977). *Handbook of Rational-Emotive Therapy.* New York: Speinges Publishing Company.

Gates-Williams, J., Jackson, M. N., Jenkins-Monroe, V. & Williams, L. R. (1992). Cross-cultural medicine: A decade later: The business of preventing African-American infant mortality. *Western Journal of Medicine,* 157, 350–356.

Gould, J. B., Davey, B. & LeRoy, S. (1989). Socioeconomic differentials and neonatal mortality; Racial comparison of California singletone. *Pediatrics,* 82 (2), 181–186.

Hogue, C. J. & Hargraves, M. A. (1993). Class, race and infant mortality in the U.S. *American Journal of Public Health,* 83 (1), 9–12.

King, L. M. (1982). Alcoholism: Studies Regarding Black Americans, 1977–1980. *Alcohol and Health Monograph 4.* Special Populations Issue, 385–407.

Laveist, T. A. (1993). Segregation, poverty and empowerment: Health concerns. *Milbank Quarterly,* 71 (1), 41–64.

Lillie-Blanton, M., MacKenzie, E. & Anthony, J. (1991). Black-white differences in alcohol use by women: Baltimore survey findings. *Public Health Reports,* 106 (2), 124–133.

Lisansky-Gomberg, E. S. & Nirenberg, T. D. (1991). Foreword: Women and substance abuse. *Journal of Substance Abuse.* 3, 131–267.

Mitchell, J. L. (1990). Low birth weight and infant mortality. *Journal of Health Social Policy,* 1 (4), 39–43.

Murray, J. L. & Bernfield, M. (1988). Differential effect of prenatal care on incidence. *New England Journal of Medicine,* 319 (21), 1385–1391.

Nichols, M. (1985). Theoretical concerns in the clinical treatment of substance-abusing women: A Feminist analysis. *Alcoholism Treatment Quarterly,* 2 (1), 79–90.

Pursley, DeWayne & Wise, Paul. (1992). Editorial: Infant mortality as a social mirror. *New England Journal of Medicine,* 326 (June 4), 1558–1560.

Russell, K. & Jewell, N. (1992). Cultural impact of health-care access: Challenges for improving the health of African-Americans. *Journal of Community Health Nursing,* 9 (3), 161–169.

Sharpe, R. & Lewis, D. (1977). *Thrive on Stress: How to Make It Work to Your Advantage.* New York: Warner Books.

Smith, R. & Draper, P. (1994). Who is in control? An investigation of nurse and patient beliefs relating to control of their health care. *Journal of Advanced Nursing,* 19, 884–892.

Stevenson, H. C. & Renard, G. (1993). Trusting ole' wise owls: Therapeutic use of cultural strengths in African-American families. *Professional Psychology: Research and Practice,* 24 (4), 433–442.

Straussner, S. L. (1985). Alcoholism in women: Current knowledge and implications for treatment. *Alcoholism Treatment Quarterly,* 2 (1), 61–75.

U.S. Bureau of the Census, Department of Commerce (1987). Money, income and poverty status of families and persons in the United States: 1986 (Advance Report). In *Current Population Reports, Consumer Income,* Series P-60, no. 157, July.

Wynne, M. J. (1985). Chitterlings, whiskey and colored folks: Chemical dependency in black Americans, an American dilemma. Unpublished manuscript.

African-American Women: Disfigured Images in the Epidemiology of Depression

Peggy Brooks-Bertram

The Johns Hopkins Hospital medical institutions were less than two blocks from my home in East Baltimore. Mothers with small children could anticipate a long wait sitting on the old wooden benches waiting to be seen in the Harriet Lane Clinic For Children. My mother and my oldest sister, sometimes serving as our mother, made this wait many times. However, my mother was also quite familiar with another clinic at Johns Hopkins, the Henry Phipps Psychiatric Clinic. The family accepted but spoke only in whispered tones about the fact that an older sister was "having problems" and needed regular psychiatric sessions for an unknown problem. The doctors said she was depressed. My mother used to explain to the neighbors and to the family that if you take a child to get a broken leg fixed, why wouldn't you take them to get their mind "fixed." While we accepted my mother's explanations, we still wondered what was wrong. If something was broken, how did it get broken? If something was broken, how was it going to get fixed? What we did know was that whatever was wrong had a profound effect on everyone.

GENERAL BACKGROUND ON DEPRESSION

Today we know much more about depression. It is a personal tragedy, as well as a major public health problem. Epidemiologic Catchment Area studies indicate an 8% lifetime prevalence for depression in the general population (Weissman, 1987). In general, depression is viewed as an affective disorder characterized by disturbances of mood. It includes negative perceptions of self such as self-blame, self-degrading unworthiness, helplessness, and hopelessness; not infrequently it includes thoughts of death or suicide (Radloff, 1980; Klerman & Weissman, 1980). It also may encompass a vegetative dimension, accompanied by loss of energy, fatigue, and impairment of bodily functioning, as reflected in disturbance of sleep, appetite, sexual interest, and gastrointestinal activity. Overall, it may result in a reduced desire and ability to execute expected roles in the family, at work, in marriage, or in school (Radloff, 1977; Klerman & Weissman, 1980). We saw all of these problems with my sister.

Depression as a condition is rather broad and can have one of three meanings: as a mood, a symptom, or a syndrome. As a mood, depression is described as part of normal sadness stemming from the general ups and downs of life. People experience such at one time or another and because these moods are short-lived, psychiatric help is generally not sought. Depression is also viewed in terms of specific symptomatology such as feeling "sad" or "blue" (Klerman & Weissman, 1980). More complicated still is the view of depression as a syndrome around which is a clustering of particular symptoms as the basis for a diagnosis of a major affective disorder.

Paykel (1991, p. 22) describes depression as "a condition in which illness shades imperceptibly through subclinical distress to a normal mood which is part of universal human experiences." Major depression, however, is the standard for classification of depression today, and is the most important diagnostic category in both ICD-10 (World Health Organization, 1992) and DSM-III-R (American Psychiatric Association, 1987) criteria. In DSM-III-R five or more specific criteria for a duration of at least two weeks are required for diagnosis (one of which must be either depressed mood or loss of interest), including depressed mood, anhedonia, significant weight loss or gain, trouble sleeping, psychomotor agitation or retardation, fatigue, feelings of worthlessness, diminished ability to think, difficulty concentrating, and suicidal thoughts.

Categories of depression include dysthymia—a chronic, less severe depression, usually with an insidious onset. Minor depression is another variant of less severe depression, and was introduced in 1978 as part of the Research Diagnostic Criteria (RCD) developed for the National Institutes of Mental Health (NIMH) Psychobiology of Depression Collaborative Study (Spitzer et al., 1978). Intermittent depression was described in the RDC as a similar diagnostic category to minor depression, but symptoms are not sustained. Recurrent brief depression was introduced by Paskin (1929). It was described as attacks of full-blown depressions that were very brief, lasting from a few hours to a few days.

Angst et al. (1990) proposed diagnostic criteria for brief recurrent depression and conducted research on its validity and described recurrent brief depression as requiring dysphoric mood or loss of interest for a duration of less than two weeks. At least four of the following must be present: poor appetite, sleep problems, agitation, loss of interest, fatigue, feelings of worthlessness, difficulty concentrating, and suicidal signs.

Another classification for depression which the DSM-IV (American Psychiatric Association, 1994) has included in its appendix is depressive personality disorder. This classification has a rather long history, and is described as excessive negative, pessimistic beliefs about oneself and others (Phillips et al., 1992). Symptoms include: (a) mood dominated by dejection, gloominess, unhappiness; (b) self-concept based on beliefs of inadequacy, worthlessness, and low self-esteem; (c) being critical, blaming, and derogatory toward oneself; (d) brooding and given to worry; (e) negativistic, critical, and judgmental toward others; (f) pessimistic; (g) prone to feeling guilt or remorse. Debate continues as to whether depressive personality disorder is separate and distinct from the other categories. Some studies show substantial overlap of these categories, particularly major depression, dysthymia, and depressive personality disorder in both nonclinical (Klein & Miller, 1993) and specialty clinical outpatient samples (Phillips et al., 1992).

While all mood disorders are found to be highly prevalent illnesses, the categories researched in community surveys include only major depression, dysthymia, and some recurrent brief depression. Individuals experience depression at various points in their life. Understanding the true prevalence of depression, especially lifetime prevalence, requires prospective, long-term epidemiological studies in which different successive age cohort samples of the general population are followed over many years. Such studies would need to take into account the numerous variables that might precipitate both the onset and recurrence of depressive disorders. These studies, though desirable, are not feasible. Thus we are left with a hodge-podge of less perfect studies covering the spectrum of anecdotal to retrospective or, less frequently prospective, epidemiological studies.

Since the landmark epidemiological studies reviewed by Boyd and Weissman (1982), a number of major epidemiological studies have been carried out in research on representative samples of the general population using various diagnostic criteria and instruments such as the Diagnostic Interview Schedule (DIS) and the Composite International Diagnostic Interview (CIDI) (Blazer & Williams, 1980; Weissman et al., 1985; Henderson, 1986; Lewinsohn et al., 1986; Bland et al., 1988; Burke et al., 1991; Robins & Reiger, 1991; Angst, 1992; Katona, 1992; Romanowski et al., 1992; Wittchen et al., 1992; Henderson et al., 1993; Kessler et al., 1994a). Wittchen et al. (1992, pp. 16–17) identified numerous other studies since 1980 that use the Research Diagnostic Criteria, the DSM-III or DSM-III-R and the ICD-10 criteria to report on the estimates of major depression,

dysthymia, and other affective disorders. They reported a number of variations as well as a point prevalence of major depression of approximately
3% (i.e., 3% of the adult population suffered from major depression at the
time of the study interview). Six-month to one-year prevalence of major
depression also varied somewhat but was approximately 6%. Wittchen et
al. also reported lifetime prevalence estimates across all the studies as
showing the most variation, with most of the recent studies reporting a
prevalence of 15–18%.

While the five-site NIMH Epidemiological Catchment Area (ECA) study
reported the lowest prevalence estimates for all time frames—for example,
lifetime prevalence of 3.0–5.9% (Robins & Reiger, 1991). Wittchen et al.
(1992) found the highest prevalence estimates resulted from studies conducted in the late 1980s or early 1990s, where at least three studies reported a prevalence range of 15–20% (Angst & Dobler-Mikola, 1985;
Wacher et al., 1992; Kessler et al., 1994a).

It is not only the high prevalence of depression that is striking, but also
the course, costs, treatment and morbidity as reflected in relapse, recurrence, comorbidity and chronicity. Studies reveal that the effects of the
morbidity of depression extends far beyond the individual. Klerman and
Weissman (1992, p. 834) for instance, broadened the scope of depression
and reviewed eight independently conducted studies. In addition to the
above problems, they report that morbidity also has an economic impact
on families and individuals which is considerable and that there is a high
social and economic burden on society. They call for future research to
completely document the effect of treatment on improving indices of economic and vocational functioning and financial independence. Special concern was also expressed for children and adolescents.

Other data on depression reveal increasing rates of prevalence. Klerman
and Weissman (1989) found that for successive birth cohorts during this
century, not only is there an increase in the prevalence of depression, but
also the age of first onset has been decreasing. Wittchen et al. (1992) cite
more recent studies in the 1990s (e.g., Cross-National Collaborative
Group, 1992; Lewinsohn et al., 1993; Kessler et al., 1994b) that address
the changing rate of major depression across the life span and findings on
temporal trends (variations in prevalence over time and can also be age,
period, or cohort trends). They report similar findings in that not only is
there an increase in the rate of prevalence of depression as well as increasing rates of depressive disorder in successively younger birth cohorts, but
also that gender differences appear to be decreasing.

Of particular note is the National Comorbidity Survey (NSC) study reporting a gender difference in cumulative onset risk that appears five years
earlier than in the ECA studies (age 10 vs. 15). The Cross-National Collaborative Group (1992) confirmed a significant trend for increasing rates
of major depression over time, in addition to an earlier age of onset for

younger cohorts. Lewinsohn et al. (1993) found a significant age-cohort effect with a trend for an earlier age of onset of illness.

Kessler et al. (1994b) in the NCS, the first survey in the United States conducted in a representative sample of the general population, found further evidence that there is a consistent trend for the lifetime risk of depression to be higher in successively younger cohorts. Another important finding of the NCS is that differences with regard to rates of depression between men and women begin in early adolescence and persist until late middle age. Burke et al. (1991) made a similar observation in the ECA studies.

If these findings are sustained in future studies, this is important because of speculation in the literature that the gender difference in depression is triggered by puberty (Nolen-Hoeksema, 1987). Puberty is reported to be a difficult emotional time for young girls, and some studies report a decrease in the age of menarche, particularly for African-American girls. Other studies report a strong relationship between age of onset of depression and risk of recurrence and chronicity (Klerman & Weissman, 1989). Clearly, Klerman and Weissman state that more research in adolescents and depression is warranted.

DEPRESSION IN WOMEN

Perhaps the most striking fact about depression is its differential sex incidence, with more women affected than men. There have been numerous studies that identify this differential. Weissman and Klerman (1977) in a review of studies between 1942 and 1973 found sex ratios (female to male) from 2.6 to 1.5 with an average female:male ratio of 2.1. In the literature as a whole there are some exceptions, but not many.

Researchers have tried to explain the sex differential through studies of help-seeking behavior (Hinkle et al., 1960; Kessler & McRae, 1981); biological causes around genes (McGuffin & Katz, 1986); hormonal differences and oral contraceptives (Weissman & Slahy, 1973); childbirth (Kendell et al., 1987; Martin et al., 1989; Dowlatshahi & Paykel, 1990); postpartum depression (Cox et al., 1989); and biological menopause (Winokur, 1973; McKinley & Jeffries, 1974; Hallstrom, 1973). Social causes as an explanation for the vast sex differential in depression have received the greatest research focus.

The studies on social explanations include life events, social support, and women's roles and status. Life event studies have shown that clinical depressions are preceded by elevated rates of the more threatening classes of life events (Paykel & Cooper, 1991). Others have shown that women react with higher symptom intensities than men to the same stress (Uhlenhuth & Paykel, 1973). Within the realm of social causes, social vulnerability studies place greater emphasis on social support. These studies are directed specifically toward women and include the seminal studies of women by Brown and Harris (1978), Brown and Prudo (1981), G. W. Brown et al. (1986). These studies address the psychosocial disadvantages of women's roles and status and report associated problems with social discrimination, inequities that lead to legal and economic helplessness, dependency on others, chronically low self-esteem, and low aspirations as factors in women's depression (G. W. Brown et al., 1986).

The epidemiological studies provide more information on women and depression. Some of these studies provided answers concerning the interactions of sex with age, marital status, and having children. The Jorm (1987) study, for example, found a curvilinear relationship between sex ratio with age and reports the female predominance most marked in middle age. Specifically, there was a high rate for women in their 20s which declined slowly as they got older. The rise in rate reached its peak well after puberty in females, and the decline started well before menopause and showed no acceleration then. This study raises questions about the relationship between an endocrine hypothesis and depression.

Gove and Tudor (1973) examined marital status and depression and found consistent trends in that high rates of mental illnesses for women are particularly accounted for by married women; single women have lower rates. For divorced, separated, and widowed women, rates are often high. They also reported that women are more detrimentally affected by marriage than men; marriage actually appears to be protective for men. In a British study, Grad de Alarcon et al. (1975), like Jorm (1987), found the expected excess of women over men in middle age, particularly for married women, as well as an excess of neurotic depression for married women aged 25–44.

Childbearing is also considered a risk factor for depression. Data on the interaction of sex with having children point in the direction of childbearing creating increased prevalence of depression. Gater et al. (1989) found that the excess in depression was accounted for by women who had one or more children. Bebbington et al. (1991) made similar observations. What is clear from these studies is that the depression peaks in women aged 20–40 who are married and have children.

It is generally agreed that women are more likely to cry easier and tend to reveal their true feelings more easily than men. Another explanation for the sex differential in depression has to do with the way in which women acknowledge their distress. Paykel (1991) suggests that women are more prepared to acknowledge their depression and to report it in surveys. Briscoe (1982) found that women are more willing to acknowledge feelings, both positive and negative. The evidence is clear that women predominate in the prevalence of depression; however, explanations for the sex differential are broad and complex and require further study, particularly in light of some recent studies reporting parity in incidence.

Data suggesting increasing rates of depression overall, concomitant with the constancy of the sex differential and earlier onset, particularly in women, is alarming. Equally distressing, and the subject of this chapter, is the near invisibility of African-American women in the study of depression in terms of both government-sponsored research as well as independent studies.

WHITE FEMINIST STUDIES OF DEPRESSION

Despite controversy over prevalence rates of depression in African-Americans and African-American women in particular (Williams, 1986; Worthington, 1992), numerous studies confirm that African-American women, representing the largest ethnic group in America, are reported to suffer disproportionately from depression. Census data provide a glimpse at the magnitude of the problem. For example, in 1988 an estimated 30.3 million African-Americans represented more than 12% of the U.S. population (U.S. Bureau of the Census, 1989a). More than 52% of that number was female, with a ratio of women to men of 110 to 100. This is in contrast to white women whose sex ratio to white males is 104 to 100. While African-American males outnumber females up to the age of 20, the number of women to men increased such that by the age of 65 the female:male ratio was a striking 149:100 (U.S. Bureau of the Census, 1989a). Some 43% of African-American households were headed by women (U.S. Bureau of the Census, 1989b), and there was an enormous disparity between the median incomes of married versus female-headed households: $27,182 and $9,710, respectively. The households with children under the age of 18 and headed by women were four times more likely to be poor than those with two-parent incomes (U.S. Bureau of the Census, 1988).

Poverty, marital status, single-parent status, and children under the age of 18 have been repeatedly identified as risk factors for depression (D. R. Brown et al., 1985). Yet there continues to be a paucity of well-designed studies of African-American women and depression. This is particularly disturbing given that the Census Tract data appear to confirm the variables that serve as the higher risk factors for African-American women and depression. To some, the status of African-American women, as reflected in the Census data, is the product of broad societal problems—namely, social injustice and inequality. And it is believed that these problems have not changed sufficiently for African-American women despite the women's movement and its advances for women in general, particularly white women.

In fact, the advent of feminism and the women's movement have not dampened African-American women's feeling of distrust and skepticism of the motives of white women in matters of women's health. For example, Audre Lorde (1984) an African-American feminist writing about African-

American women's health, described white feminists as "tools of the master" (p. 112) who could not be expected to dismantle the master's house. Further she states that

if white American feminist theory need not deal with the differences between us, and the resulting differences in our oppressions, then how do you deal with the fact that the women who clean your houses and tend your children while you attend conferences on feminist theory are, for the most part, poor women and women of color? What is the theory behind racist feminism" (p. 112)?

Angela Davis (1983) discussed the barriers black women faced from white women during the early women's movement. For instance, African-American women were barred access into abolitionist groups and women's rights organizations. Still others believed that African-American women were the principal targets of racism and sexism (Beale, 1970).

If the recent U.S. Census data are any indication, most African-Americans would believe that African-American women remain the targets of racism and sexism (U.S. Bureau of the Census, 1988). Ladner (1973, p. xiii) advised that a "frontal attack" must be made on the myths of black womanhood as much as against "hunger and . . . brutality. Ultimately, all of these injustices are interdependent." As bell hooks (1981, pp. 7–8) has pointed out, "when black people are talked about, sexism militates against the acknowledgment of the interests of black women; when women are talked about racism militates against a recognition of black women's interest."

The purpose of this chapter, therefore, is to identify and review studies on African-American women and depression. And because of the landmark studies of women and depression conducted by white feminist psychologists, it is important to begin this examination by looking at these early efforts and understanding their impact on the paucity of studies of African-American women and depression. In fact, a paper on the literature on African-American women and depression would be remiss if it did not address the role of white feminists in studying depression as a discrete psychiatric condition and its contribution to the paucity of studies specifically addressing depression and African-American women. There is no question but that white feminists had an enormous influence on both psychotherapy and psychiatry, especially regarding depression. This research originally emerged to challenge a male bias that has existed for many years. But it is safe to say that this advance left as casualties African-American women and, indeed, other women of color.

The near absence of African-American women in studies of depression is quite evident. And, despite broad literature on depression, particularly depression and women, there remains a paucity of studies directed specifically to African-American women. This remains true despite numerous studies identifying greater prevalence of depression among African-American women compared to all other groups across the age spectrum. This continuing paucity requires an examination of issues that speak to the broader societal problems of racism and other social injustices experienced by African-American women.

In this light, white feminists' approaches to the identification of the etiology of depression in women are critical to this discussion. Feminists, for example, had an enormous influence on psychotherapy, particularly for women, and the study of depression in women and contributed to a number of issues, (e.g., treatment of depression) and to the development of therapist variables such as effects of therapist, process, and client dimensions (McGrath et al., 1993). Later, sex bias in psychotherapy was also examined. The decade of the 1970s was ushered in with feminist studies of the demographics of psychotherapy: These studies found that therapists are mostly male, whereas their clients are mostly female; and that the longest treatment relationships are most likely to be between attractive young male therapists and attractive young female clients (Chesler 1972; Gove & Tudor, 1973). Chesler (1972), for example, provided the impetus for clinical researchers to examine assessment and treatment issues.

With all of these forward-moving steps in the mental health of women, there was also backward motion for African-American women and depression. It appears that in the white feminists' march forward in the study of depression, they excluded other women, thereby maintaining and reinforcing socially constructed concepts of a hierarchical social order—the basis of racism and white supremacy—in the study of depression in women.

In the early feminist studies of women and depression, African demonstration of feminists' view of African-American women is that expressed in the groundbreaking feminist study of women and depression by Chesler (1972). This work became an impetus for clinical researchers to examine assessment and treatment issues, particularly in depression. Chesler (p. 2), however, opens her work with the statement:

I have no theory to offer to Third World female psychology in America. No single theory will do descriptive justice to women of African, Latin-American, Mexican, Chinese, and native Indian descent. Furthermore, as a white woman, I'm reluctant and unable to construct theories about experiences I haven't had . . . as a psychologist and feminist, I am really more interested in exploring the laws of female psychology than in exploring their various exceptions and variations.

It is clear in this statement that not only was Chesler's reference to other women as Third World demeaning, but she also made a clear distinction between the psychology of white women and that of other women, thereby relegating the psychology of other women to the lesser status of "exceptions and variations." Second, her words implied that it was only "descriptive justice" (as opposed to in-depth analysis) that African, Latin-American, Mexican, Chinese, and women of native Indian descent warranted or could hope to attain. Third, she was not only unwilling to construct theories about other womens' experiences but was unable to see possibilities for theory development in what some of these other women had already written about themselves. Nor could she see how these writings could be significant for the study of these women's depressions. Finally, and most important, she defined a hierarchy within female psychology: laws were attributed to white female psychology while variations, exceptions, and, implicitly, deviations, were applied to all others.

This assignment of hierarchy appeared to be based on racial distinction and was not unlike that described by Thomas and Sillen (1972) in a work on racism in psychiatry. They identified two basic themes in white racism: that black people are born with inferior brains and a limited capacity for mental growth, and that their personality tends to be abnormal. Thomas and Sillen viewed these concepts of inferiority and pathology as both interrelated and reinforcing. Both "have served to sanctify a hierarchical social order" (p. 13).

The continuation of "social hierarchies" is most regrettable in feminist studies of depression because the Chesler work is regarded by many as an outstanding landmark study, despite its serious limitations with regard to nonwhite women. From a feminist perspective, it explores the realities behind women's careers (white middle-class women) as psychiatric patients. It also identifies sex-role stereotyping as a key factor in mental illness. Chesler also exposed the perpetuation of violence against women within psychiatry. Again, regrettably, it appears that the initial designation of a white and nonwhite psychology in this groundbreaking study of depression signaled a research course characterized by the stymieing of research into the etiology, course, diagnosis, and treatment of depression in African-American women.

In a study of social class and psychiatric disturbance among women in an urban population, G. W. Brown et al. (1975, p. 248) state that "certain groups of women in our society have a significantly greater than average risk of suffering from depressive conditions to the extent that the unequal distribution of such risk is the result of more widely recognized inequities within our society . . . we believe that it constitutes a major social injustice." This is certainly true for African-American women and it is why the impact of the feminist hierarchical approach to studying depression is so devastating to research on African-American women. In fact, the effect is clear across the broad space of studies in the depression of women, whether they are studies of discrete conditions, ECA studies, or other epidemiologic studies.

STUDIES OF AFRICAN-AMERICAN WOMEN AND DEPRESSION

Despite early and indeed continuing neglect, researchers are slowly trying to rectify both the paucity and invisibility of African-American women in the literature of depression (Barbee, 1992; Jackson, 1993). Others (Williams, 1986) are concerned with the biases generated from studies that rely on data gathered from only poor, socially disadvantaged African-American women. This section will identify the literature, although the listings are incomplete. Before discussing the literature, it is important to identify community surveys as an important source of data on African-American mental health in general, despite the problems of conducting this research with African-Americans.

Depression has been researched in African-Americans, mostly through treatment studies and early community surveys. That literature is treated more extensively in Neighbors (1984) and D. R. Brown et al. (1985) and will not be reviewed here. Survey research, however, is the more prominent method of discerning discrete psychiatric conditions (e.g., depression), but not without concern. For example, researchers have criticized the appropriateness of using survey research in African-American communities (Myers, 1979). Others express concern because of several problems that may result in response bias as well as problems with inaccurate data (Worthington, 1992). Still others have identified the difficulties of conducting large-scale surveys in minority communities (Milburn et al., 1991).

Surveys remain the most widely used technique for collecting social science data because a variety of information can be collected from large samples at reasonable costs (Barbee, 1973). Milburn et al. (1991) identify the difficulties of conducting surveys in minority communities as including low response rates, interviewer bias, and the development of adequate sampling strategies to tap diverse segments within minority communities and locate specific segments of the population, such as male respondents (p. 3). Despite these problems, surveys have been successful in gathering information about the prevalence of depression. Milburn et al. caution that researchers can and have identified these problems and structured the surveys to overcome them. For instance, response rate has been a major problem in surveying the African-American community.

However, response rates in several surveys of African-American communities have ranged from 67 to 74%, indicating that good response rates are obtainable (Dressler & Badger, 1985; Gary et al., 1984, 1989; Neighbors & Jackson 1986). Each of these surveys addresses depression or psychological distress in African-American communities. Achieving sociodemographic heterogeneity in African-American samples has also been a problem. The work of Dressler (1985), Gary et al. (1984), and Neighbors and Jackson (1986) emphasizes the need for diversity in the African-American population under study.

There is, however, a growing body of literature, albeit limited, which speaks specifically to depression in African-American women. This is particularly important in light of the continuing depressing economic outlook for African-American women reflected in U.S. Census statistics. First, there have been a number of reviews of the literature on specific topics addressing African-Americans and mental illness, including the epidemiology of mental illness in African-Americans (Neighbors & Lumpkin, 1990); psychiatric morbidity in African-Americans (Neighbors, 1984); improving African-American mental health in general (Neighbors, 1987); and depression (D. R. Brown, 1990).

Williams (1986) reviewed epidemiologic studies of mental illness in African-Americans, emphasizing problems with the NIMH ECA studies. Of particular relevance is Williams' suggestion that because the current ECA reports do not clearly state the degree to which reported survey findings for African-Americans are based upon a sample of predominantly poor, urban African-American females, there is the distinct possibility that the findings for this subpopulation will be used to define rates of psychiatric illness for all African-Americans, regardless of their class or gender. Other points of particular importance Williams also suggests are that there has been a shift away from the health needs of African-Americans to those of the Hispanic population (p. 48). Williams stated that the ECA studies, while a major advance in communitywide field studies of whites, are seriously flawed and misleading as a national survey of mental illness in African-Americans (p. 48). He attributes this in part to the fact that these studies have also failed to obtain a statistically significant sampling of middle- and upper-income African-Americans, thereby making generalizability of findings to all African-Americans difficult if not impossible.

Others have conducted reviews that identified specific issues. For instance, Worthington (1992) reviewed the literature on emphasizing the factors influencing the diagnosis and treatment of African-American patients in the mental health system (e.g., racial and ethnic factors as they pertain to the misdiagnosis of the African-American client). This review identified important questions about cultural relativism theory and labeling theory regarding nurses and lay African-American views on problematic behavior of African-American patients. In particular it identified an absence of difference in labeling behavior between black and white nurses—a finding that Worthington views as presenting new questions about African-American health professionals adopting and applying to African-American patients the stereotypes of white professionals. She stresses the need for more research on this finding. Worthington also reports that most researchers found diagnostic and treatment differences related to race (p. 202); that ethnocentric concepts that depression is infrequent in African-Americans is dispelled; and that differential responses between whites and African Americans needs further study.

Barbee (1992) also provides a review and critique of the literature on American women and depression. Both the Worthington and Barbee reviews appear to represent the only literature reviews specifically addressing African-American women and depression. Interestingly enough, both are found in the psychiatric nursing literature and were conducted by nurses. Barbee emphasizes the absence of "special sensitivity" (p. 257) and the lack of contextual research with African-American women and depression. She examines these issues with reference to the assessment, diagnoses, treatment, and prevention of mental health problems in African-American women. Citing Olmedo and Parron (1981), she reports that professionals still know very little about minority women; there continues to be an absence of reliable systematic data on population size; quality of data on the epidemiology of mental disorders among African-American women is lacking; data on a number of aspects of help-seeking behavior for mental health services is lacking; there is a failure to acknowledge the heterogeneity of minority women; and there is evidence of the perpetuation of myths about minority women derived from anecdotal literature.

Barbee (1992) describes these studies as exhibiting little special sensitivity to African-American women, "acontextual," and lacking in understanding of how African-American women live their lives (p. 257). She discusses issues of racism and European-American psychiatry and distinguishes between "acontextual depression research" (p. 259) which she asserts essentially ignores the reality of African-American women's experiences with depression. On the other hand, contextual depression research is described as research that tries to discover why African-American women feel the way they do, discovers their true feelings and understands why they feel the way they do, and tries to identify mechanisms to help them feel better. She identifies several studies as contextual (Dressler & Badger, 1985; Dressler, 1985) which report, respectively, that greater symptoms for women were modified by community and geography and that there was a positive relationship between local region and support and depressive symptoms. Barbee expressed concern that despite the evidence for contextual research, acontextual research dominates the literature (p. 260). For example, in her critique of scales frequently used in depression research with African-Americans, Barbee identifies scales that found a large number of African-American women at risk for or in need of treatment for depression, for example, scales utilized by (Radloff, 1977). She asserts that a major failing was that all of the data presented by Radloff was based on Euro-American groups. Further, she reports that one study using cross-validation of self-report measures of depression found it easier for some cultural groups to endorse a particular symptom's frequency or intensity than it was to report a mood. The symptom frequency endorsement appeared to produce higher depression scores than symptom intensity and mood description measures. In her own work with samples consisting of African-American women only, Barbee (1992) found that African-American women described themselves as depressed based on both the duration of intensity of symptoms and the extent to which normal activities and relationships were disrupted. These are very important distinctions that should be researched further in larger heterogeneous studies.

Barbee (1992) also critiques the Epidemiological Catchment Area studies. While these are viewed as some of the most important studies of depression in community settings, she considers them to be acontextual and concludes that there is limited literature devoted to the treatment of depressed African-American women. Major complaints on existing literature include: failure of researchers to examine the interactive effects of risks for African-American women and depression; limited studies of primary prevention efforts; failure to identify racism, sexism, and classism as key factors in depression in African-American women; and sparse attention to the risks of depression to middle-income and professional African-American women, thereby limiting the study of intraethnic diversity and depression. Barbee's suggestions include a call for research that explores the interactions among gender, race, class, and depression. This is a very important review of the literature from the perspective of American women.

MIXED SAMPLES OF DEPRESSION IN AFRICAN-AMERICANS

There are also a number of studies directed specifically toward African-Americans utilizing both male and female subjects. Dressler (1985), for example, found in a study of social supports and mental health in a southern black community that for females over the age of 34, extended kin support is associated with fewer symptoms of depression by about the same magnitude as economic stressors are related to a larger number of symptoms. Dressler reports that a puzzling finding was that young women aged 17–34 perceive the higher level of extended kin support and yet report the greatest number of depressive symptoms (p. 45). Dressler concludes that other processes are at work.

In a study of manic-depressive illness among poor urban blacks, Jones et al. (1981) found that manic-depressive illness does occur among low-socioeconomic blacks and at a rate that is significant and warrants further research. The manic-depressive group was relatively young, there were 3.5 times as many women as men, and more than half of the group had been married at some time. Neighbors (1983) conducted a major study on help-seeking behavior in African-Americans, utilizing a national sample of adult African-Americans. It was designed to elucidate help-seeking behavior of African-Americans for mental health services. The sample resulted in 2,107 completed interviews, with a response rate of 67%. Oddly enough, this study made no specific mention of African-American female use of mental health services.

Dressler and Badger (1985), in a study of the epidemiology of depressive symptoms in three black communities, suggest that young females and males in various marital statuses should be followed over time in order to determine more precisely the stressors and resistance resources that most directly influence the risk of depression. They also found that mean symptoms and rates of high depressive symptoms were higher among women, younger persons, divorced and separated persons, and unemployed persons, thereby corroborating findings of earlier studies.

AFRICAN-AMERICAN WOMEN COMPARED WITH OTHER ETHNIC GROUPS

Although research cites the high prevalence rates of depression among African-American women, that evidence does not appear to have sparked major research interest in depression in African-American women. On the other hand, there are numerous studies of comparisons of African-American women with other minorities, such as Native Americans, Mexicans and others (Quesada et al., 1978; Caste et al., 1978). Interestingly enough, in these studies the cultural differences on these groups are highlighted while those of African-American women are minimized or ignored. Even when compared to other minority women, African-American women are found to predominate in prevalence of depression. In a study of young Asian, African-American, and white women in the United States, for example, it was found that of the three groups of women aged 18–45, African-American women had the greatest number of children, the lowest education and income, the greatest number of negative and positive life events, and the smallest unconflicted network size. All of these variables have been found to place women at high risk for depression. And for African-American women, the number of negative life events, conflicted network size, and low religiosity were associated with higher depression scores (Woods et al., 1994).

Additionally, although greater interest has been shown in depression as a discrete psychiatric illness among other ethnic groups—for example, Asian Indian women (Jambunathan, 1992), Hispanic women (Amaro et al., 1987), culture and depression in married Mexican immigrant women (Salgado de Snyder, 1987), Mexican women and traditional cultural expectations and predisposition to depression (Hernandez, 1986), acculturation of Puerto Ricans in the United States (Comas-Diaz, 1981), acculturation and psychopathology among Puerto Rican women in mainland United States (Torres-Matrullo, 1976), cross-cultural studies of Native Americans (Shore et al., 1987), Indo-Chinese women (Kleinman, 1980), and Laotian refugees (Davidson-Muskilhn et al., 1989)—there remain a very limited number of studies of African-American women and depression. This incomplete number of studies seems to corroborate Williams' (1986) assertion that interest in the health of African-Americans has shifted to that of other ethnic groups, particularly Hispanics. This may have negative implications for researching depression in African-American women.

Stress is also related to depression and the literature on stress and African-American women is extensive but will not be reviewed here. However, it should be pointed out that black women are exposed to excessive and probably more frequent stressors than are their white counterparts. Black women's stresses are viewed to be an outgrowth of cultural, structural, and most likely discriminatory experiences (Kessler, 1979).

STUDIES OF SELF-HELP FOR AFRICAN-AMERICANS

Although a 1990 report on women and depression from the American Psychological Association (APA) concluded that women of color are at greater risk for depression than any other group (McGrath et al., 1990), it is painfully evident that only small effort has been made in this area. Exceptions include Barbee (1994) and Jackson (1993). In a study specifically addressing depression in African-American women, Barbee (1994) presented findings from a unique, though small, study that examined how African-American women identified depression and dysphoric mood states and their techniques of self-help in each state. Barbee reported that this group of women described the two states quite differently from mental health professionals' descriptions of dysphoria as a pathological healing state. In fact, her subjects considered "the blues" as a transition mood between feeling down. On the other hand, they viewed depression as the signal that they needed time for themselves.

Barbee (1994) also found that these women identified two subtypes of the blues and their coping strategies for each also differed. For instance, when experiencing "mild blues," they employed solitary, self-consoling activities. When they identified the "blues" as severe, they reported seeking assistance in spiritual, interpersonal, and solitary activities, such as reading the Bible or engaging with friends. Overall, these women found the "blues" to have regenerative qualities because it facilitated introspective and spiritual renewal.

While a number of questions can be raised about this study, it is especially important because of its cultural specificity—for example, even employing culturally relevant descriptors, like "the blues," so as to help the study sample more adequately describe their feelings. Most surprising is the finding that African-American women did not particularly find depressive and dysphoric mood states as all bad or dysfunctional. Certainly self-help techniques of African-American women in depression require further investigation.

Jackson (1993) examined the relationship between depression and income, education, age, social support, marital status, attitude toward mate, and role strain in African-American women. While these risk factors have been studied extensively by other researchers, they have not been examined solely in the context of African-American women and depression. Jackson utilized a sample of women who were economically diverse. This economic diversity is important because criticisms (Williams, 1986) have been launched about the effect of the predominance of low-economic women in fear of attempts to generalize the findings from those samples to the general population. Jackson reports that the best predictors for depression were younger women with less marital satisfaction and low income. On the other hand, unmarried women with less social support and more role strain reported more depression. There is a need to examine the interactive effects of these risks. Others assert that "the assessment, diagnoses, treatment, and prevention of mental health problems in minority women require special sensitivity" (Barbee, 1992, p. 257).

CONCLUSIONS

This work represents neither a complete review of the literature on African-American women and depression nor of the entire body of depression research that includes African-American women in the samples. It does, however, indicate that an understanding of African-American women and depression can be gleaned only through a rather eclectic literature representing a mixture of literature reviews, specific studies of African-American women, community surveys not specific to African-American women, epidemiological studies of national samples of African-Americans to determine the prevalence of mental illness, studies of depression with comparisons of African-American women with other ethnic women groups, general discussions on approaches to mental health for African-Americans, and studies of comparisons of African-Americans in general with other ethnic groups.

While this eclecticism is a reflection of considerable effort, research on African-American women and depression could probably best be described as having been thwarted by attention to white women and depression with the attendant effect of little attention to the agony of depression in other women, especially African-American women. It also appears to represent an unguided, shotgun approach to the study of depression in African-American women.

What is clearly missing, therefore, is the type of concerted and sustained effort begun in the 1970s by feminist psychologists and psychiatrists, who first began examination of white women and mental illness (namely, depression) but which excluded African-American women primarily by virtue of white feminists' choice of white male patriarchy as the oppressor of white women, while at the same time excluding racism, sexism, and classism as the oppressors of African-American women. What is needed is a culturally specific theory postulating the etiology of depression in African-American women.

IMPLICATIONS AND RECOMMENDATIONS
FOR FURTHER RESEARCH

More than 20 years after the first groundbreaking study of depression in white women, studies of African-American women and depression are being conducted, albeit slowly. There is considerable ground to make up in recovering from the early feminists' perpetuation of the notion of separate psychology for white and African-American women. Gender-related, societal, and cultural conditions compound risk factors for depression in African-American women. It is firmly established, though not without continuing questions, that certain risk factors place African-American women at risk for greater prevalence of depression and that they suffer, according to most studies, disproportionately, particularly in the middle years. Therefore it is now imperative that researchers revisit the "scene of the crime," if you will, and begin to build from scratch culturally relevant theories of the causation, course, and treatment of depression in African-American women.

Researchers should not hesitate to cast a broad net in identifying and/or developing theories, particularly those that seek to explore the physical and emotional consequences of social inequality. Ussher (1993, p. 298) puts it aptly: "we need to look to the individual woman's needs, her personal path to misery, and offer help accordingly. But we also need to attack the underlying structures and institutions which perpetuate women's oppression." Mental health research, specifically that designed to understand depression in African-American women, must be structured to reflect knowledge of, and sensitivity to, the effects of continuing social inequality. While we have a preponderance of data on risk factors about depression, we still know very little about the mechanisms by which these factors contribute either singly or interactively to cause. The studies reviewed thus far, while in no way reflecting the complete literature, represent a patchwork of efforts to assess, diagnose, and treat depression in African-American women.

What is needed is a focused research approach identifying a specific variable, much as the feminists identified patriarchy and gender. They continue to examine various dimensions of aspects of both. Studies of African-American women and depression also need to reflect a construct—

racism—and to build the research on African-American women and depression around the mechanisms by which racism creates and contributes to depression in these women. Feminists ignored racism as a component in their earlier paradigms of depression in women. There is also a need to move beyond risk-factor identification and to develop theories on the pathways by which these factors result in depression. A theory is needed not only to guide the construction of studies that reflect both the lived experiences of African-American women in the United States but also to identify the nuances of the culture that guide those experiences. African-American researchers, especially, should be more aggressive in designing theories that allow them to more adequately explain the etiology, course, and dimensions of depression.

Depression is not going to go away. Instead, there is substantial evidence indicating increasing rates of depression (Klerman & Weissman, 1989, p. 2229.) This has serious implications for African-American women as a whole, particularly for younger women. Klerman and Weissman report that the data suggest that across the health care spectrum there are greater numbers and younger patients presenting with major depression, either alone or with a comorbid physical illness and its complications. They recommend the use of longitudinal designs with repeated assessment of the psychiatric state of successive births to facilitate ongoing surveillance of the increase. Because any of these efforts will involve considerable funding, it is especially imperative that funding be identified to study depression in African-American women as they are a seriously underresearched group that is at disproportionate risk for depression.

In a study of the research funding of mental illness and addictive disorders, Pincus and Fine (1992) stated that despite the undeniable and substantial toll on human life and productivity, the level of research support for these disorders is extremely limited and disproportionate to the overall costs to society by these disorders. In terms of the best avenues for funding, the study findings underscore the preeminence of the NIMH, the National Institute on Drug Abuse, and the National Institute on Alcohol Abuse and Alcoholism in the conduct of mental illness, substance abuse, and psychiatric research. Pincus and Fine mentioned a study of these agencies which indicates that they provide 76% of all sources of research support (p. 578). It therefore seems reasonable to suggest that it is to these agencies that researchers need to turn to finance research on African-American women and depression. Perhaps a most likely candidate is the NIMH, which, through its Epidemiological Catchment Area studies, has previously shown a commitment to estimating the prevalence of mental illness in large populations across the country as well as the development of culturally sensitive diagnostic tools such as the Diagnostic Interview Schedule modified for African-Americans (Hendricks et al., 1983). Nonetheless, shrinking research funds (Pincus & Fine 1992), increasing rates of depression (Klerman & Weissman, 1989) are disturbing, particularly for African-American women because the combination of increasing rates of depression with a corresponding decrease in the age of first onset (Fombonne, 1994) and with age of first onset as a predictor for recurrent depression (Klerman & Weissman, 1989), as well as some researchers' belief that there has been a shift away from the health needs of African-Americans to that of the Hispanic population (Williams, 1986), is indeed a deadly combination and portends continued and unnecessary suffering for African-American women.

African-American women and depression is clearly one of the most neglected and most-needed areas of research in mental health. Investigators, as attested to by the paucity of studies with this population, have only just begun to approach the problem of depression and African-American women. Particularly puzzling is the emergence of the study of African-American women and depression via psychiatric nursing instead of psychiatry.

Recommendations for the future of this research should include the mechanisms by which the consequences of racial inequality translate into depression in African-American women. There is a need for:

- constructing depression as a physical/emotional consequence of social inequality
- examination of the heterogeneity of both shared and unique experiences within African-American women as a group and their relationship with depression
- examination of gender and ethnic stereotyping in the therapeutic relationship and its role in the treatment of depression
- continued work on ascertaining the appropriateness of current diagnostic categories and assessment instruments for identifying depression in African-American women
- investigation of the interactive effects of risk factors for the various dimensions of depression by age, occupation, education, income, and health status
- examination of differential responses to various types of treatment across groups
- identification of correlation among depression and other conditions such as eating disorders and substance abuse in African-American women
- investigation of African-American women's perceptions of what constitutes depression and what is the "blues"
- isolating the mechanisms that link sociodemographic factors to increased depression in African-American women because of the divergent age patterns of risk

WORKS CITED

Amaro, H., Russo, N. F. & Johnson, J. (1987). Family and work predictors of psychological well-being among Hispanic women professionals. *Psychology of Women Quarterly*, 11, 502–522.

American Psychiatric Association. (1987). *Diagnostic and Statistical Manual of*

Mental Disorders, 3rd ed, rev. (DSM-III-R). Washington, DC: American Psychiatric Association.

American Psychiatric Association. (1994). *Diagnostic and Statistical Manual of Mental Disorders,* 4th ed. (DSM-IV). Washington, DC: American Psychiatric Association.

Angst, J. (1992). Epidemiology of depression. *Psychopharmacology,* 106, S71–S74.

Angst, J. & Dobler-Mikola, A. (1985). The Zurich study: VI A continuum from depression to anxiety disorders. *European Archives of Psychiatry and Neurological Sciences,* 23, 179–186.

Angst, J., Merikangas, K., Schneidegger, P. et al. (1990). Recurrent brief depression, a new subtype of depressive disorder. *Journal of Affective Disorders,* 19, 87–98.

Barbee, E. (1973). *Survey Research Methods.* Belmont, CA: Wadsworth.

Barbee, E. (1984). Healing time: The blues and African American women. *Health Care for Women International,* 15, 53–60.

Barbee E. L. (1992). African American women and depression: A review and critique of the literature. *Archives of Psychiatric Nursing,* 7 (5), 257–265.

Beale, Francis. (1970). Double jeopardy in the black woman. In Toni Cade, ed., *The Black Woman.* New York: Mentor/New American Library, p. xiii.

Bebbington, P. E., Dean, C., Der, G. et al. (1991). Gender, parity and the prevalence of minor affective disorder. *British Journal of Psychiatry,* 158, 40–45.

Bland, R. C., Orn, H., and Newman, S. E. (1988). Lifetime prevalence of psychiatric disorders in Edmonton. *Acta Psychiatria Scandinavica* Suppl 338, 77: 24–32.

Blazer, D. & Williams, C. D. (1980). Epidemiology of dysphoria and depression in an elderly population. *American Journal of Psychiatry,* 137, 439–444.

Boyd, J. H. & Weissman, M. M. (1982). Epidemiology. In E. S. Paykel, ed., *Handbook of Affective Disorders.* Edinburgh: Churchhill Livingstone, 109–115.

Brisco, M. (1982). Sex Differences in Psychological Well-Being. *Psychological Medicine* (Monograph Suppl. 1), 10.

Brown, D. R. (1990). Depression among Blacks: An Epidemiologic Perspective. In D. S. Ruiz, ed., *Handbook of Mental Health and Mental Disorder Among Black Americans.* Westport, CT: Greenwood Press, 71–91.

Brown, D. R. et al. (1985). Predictors of depressive symptoms among unemployed black adults. *Journal of Sociology and Social Welfare,* 12, 736–750.

Brown, G. W., Andrews, B. & Harris, T. O. et al. (1986). Social support, self-esteem and depression. *Psychological Medicine,* 16, 813–831.

Brown, G. W., Bhrolchain, D. & Harris, T. O. (1975). Social class and psychiatric disturbance among women in an urban population. *Sociology,* 9 (2), 225–254.

Brown, G. W. & Harris, T. O. (1978). *Social Origins of Depression: A Study of Psychiatric Disorder in Women.* London: Tavistock.

Brown, G. W. & Prudo, R. (1981). Psychiatric disorder in a rural and an urban population. *Psychological Medicine,* 11, 581–599.

Burke, K. C., Burke, J. D., Rae, D. S. et al. (1991). Comparing age at onset of major depression and other psychiatric disorders by birth cohorts in five U.S. community populations. *Archives of General Psychiatry,* 48, 789–795.

Caste, C., Blodgett, J. & Rubinow, D. (1978). Cross-cultural differences in presenting problems: Implications for service delivery and treatment modality. Unpublished manuscript, Yale University School of Medicine, Department of Psychiatry.

Chesler, P. (1972). *Women and Madness.* New York: Doubleday.

Comas-Diaz, L. (1981). Effects of cognitive and behavioral group treatment in the depressive symptomatology of Puerto Rican women. *Journal of Counseling Clinical Psychology,* 49, 627–632.

Cox, J. L., Paykel, E. S. & Page, M. L. (1989). Current Approaches: Childbirth as a Life Event. *Southampton Duphar Medical Relations.*

Cross-National Collaborative Group. (1992). The changing rate of major depression: cross-national comparisons. *The Journal of the American Medical Association,* 268, 3098–3105.

Davidson-Muskilhn, M. & Golden, C. (1989). Lao depression inventory. *Journal of Personality Assessment,* 53, 161–168.

Davis, A. (1983). *Women, Race and Class.* New York: Random House.

Dowlatshahi, D. & Paykel, E. S. (1990). Life events and social stress in puerperal psychosis: absence of effect. *Psychological Medicine,* 20, 655–662.

Dressler, W. W. (1985). Extended family relationships, social supports and mental health in a Southern black community. *Journal of Health and Social Behavior,* 26, 39–48.

Dressler, W. W. & Badger, L. W. (1985). Epidemiology of depressive symptoms in black communities: A comparative analysis. *Journal of Nervous and Mental Disease,* 173, 212–220.

Fombonne, E. (1994). Increased rates of depression: Update of epidemiological findings and analytical problems. *Acta Psychiatrica Scandinavica,* 90, 145–156.

Gary, L. E. et al. (1984). *Pathways: A Study of Black Informal Network Supports,* Final report. Washington, DC: Howard University, Institute for Urban Affairs and Research.

Gary, L. E. et al. (1989). *Depression in Black American Adults: Findings from the Norfolk Area Health Study,* Final Report. Washington, DC: Howard University, Institute for Urban Affairs and Research.

Gater, R. A., Dean, C. & Morris, J. (1989). The contribution of childbearing to the sex difference in first admission rates for affective psychoses. *Psychological Medicine,* 19, 719–724.

Gove, W. R. & Tudor, J. R. (1973). Adult sex roles and mental illness. *American Journal of Sociology,* 78, 812–835.

Grad de Alarcon, J., Sainsbury, P. & Costain, W. R. (1975). Incidence of referred mental illness in Chichester and Salisbury. *Psychological Medicine,* 5, 32–54.

Hallstrom, T. (1973). *Mental Disorder and Sexuality in the Climacteric.* Goteberg, Sweden: Ortadius Biktryckeri AB.

Henderson, A. S. (1986). Epidemiology of mental illness. In H. Hafner, G. Moschel & N. Sartorius, eds., *Mental Health in the Elderly: A Review of the Present State of Research.* Berlin: Springer, 29–34.

Henderson, A. S., Jorm, A. F. & MacKinnon, A. (1993). The prevalence of depressive disorders and the distribution of depressive symptoms in later life:

a survey using draft ICD-10 and DSM-III-R. *Psychological Medicine, 23,* 719–729.

Hendricks, L., Bayton, J., Collins, J., Mathura, C., McMillan, S. & Montgomery, T. (1983). NIMH's Diagnostic Interview Schedule: A test of its concurrent validity in a population of black adults. *Journal of the National Medical Association, 75,* 667–671.

Hernandez, M. (1986). Depression among Mexican Women: A transgenerational perspective. Paper presented at the biannual meeting of the National Coalition of Hispanic Health and Human Services Organization, New York.

Hinkle, L. E, Redmont, R., Plummer, N. et al. (1960). An explanation of the relation between symptoms, disability and serious illness in two homogeneous groups of men and women. *Journal of Public Health, 50,* 1327–1336.

hooks, bell (1981). *Aint I a Woman: Black Women and Feminism.* Boston: South End Press.

Jackson, M. (1993). Factors related to depression in African-American women. Unpublished Dissertation, University of Cincinnati.

Jambunathan, J. (1992). Sociocultural factors in depression in Asian Indian Women. *Health Care for Women International, 13,* 261–270.

Jones, B. E., Gray, B. A. & Parson, E. (1981). Manic depressive illness among poor urban blacks. *American Journal of Psychiatry, 138* (5), 654–657.

Jorm, A. F. (1987). Sex and age differences in depression: a quantitative synthesis of published research. *Australian and New Zealand Journal of Psychiatry, 21,* 46–53.

Katona, C. L. (1992). The epidemiology of depression in old age: The importance of physical illness. *Clinical Neuropharmacology, 15* (suppl.), 281A–282A.

Kendell, R. E., Chalmers, J. C. & Platz, C. (1987). Epidemiology of puerperal psychoses. *British Journal of Psychiatry, 150,* 662–673.

Kessler, J. R. (1979). Stress, social status and psychological distress. *Journal of Health and Social Behavior, 20,* 259–272.

Kessler, R. C., McGonagle, K. A., Zhao, S. et al. (1994a). Lifetime and 12-month prevalence of DSM-III-R psychiatric disorders in the U.S.: Results from the National Comorbidity Survey. *Archives of General Psychiatry, 51,* 8–19.

Kessler, R. C., McGonagle, K. A., Nelson, C. B. et al. (1994b). Sex and depression in the National Comorbidity Survey II: Cohort effects. *Journal of Affective Disorders, 30,* 15–26.

Kessler, R. C. & McRae, J. A., Jr. (1981). Trends in the relationship between sex and psychological distress: 1957–1976. *American Sociological Review, 46,* 443–452.

Klein, D. M. & Miller, G. A. (1993). Depressive personality in a non-clinical sample. *American Journal of Psychiatry, 150,* 1718–1724.

Kleinman, A. (1980). *Patients and Healers in the Context of Culture.* Berkeley: University of California Press.

Klerman, G. & Weissman, M. (1980). Depressions among women: Their nature and causes. In M. Gutentag, ed. *The Mental Health of Women.* New York: Academic Press.

Klerman, G. L. & Weissman, M. M. (1992). The course, morbidity, and costs of depression. *Archives of General Psychiatry, 49,* 831–834.

Klerman, G. L. & Weissman, M. M. (1989). Increasing rates of depression. *Journal of the American Medical Association*, 261, 2229–2235.

Ladner, Joyce. (1973). Foreword to Robert Staples, *The Black Woman in America: Sex, Marriage and the Family*. Chicago: Nelson-Hall.

Lewinsohn, P. M., Duncan, E. M., Stanton, A. K. et al. (1986). Age at first onset for nonbipolar depression. *Journal of Abnormal Psychology*, 95, 378–383.

Lewinsohn, P. M., Rohde, P., Seeley, J., Fischer, S. A. (1993). Age cohort changes in the lifetime occurrence of depression and other mental disorders. *Journal of Abnormal Psychology*, 102 (1), 110–120.

Lorde, Audre. (1984). *Sister Outsider: Essays and Speeches by Audre Lorde*. Freedom, CA: The Crossing Press.

Martin, C. J., Brown, G. W., Goldberg, D. P. et al. (1989). Psychosocial stress and puerperal depression. *Journal of Affective Disorders*, 16, 283–293.

McGrath, E., Keita, G. P., Strickland, B. R. & Russo, N. F. (1993). *Women and Depression: Risk Factors and Treatment Issues*. Final Report of the American Psychological Association National Task Force on Women and Depression. Washington, DC: American Psychological Association, 41–73.

McGuffin, R. & Katz, R. (1986). Nature, nurture and affective disorder. In J. F. W. Deakin, ed., *The Biology of Depression*. London: Royal College of Psychiatrists.

McKinley, S. M. & Jeffries, M. (1974). The menopausal syndrome. *British Journal of Preventive and Social Medicine*, 28, 108–115.

Milburn, N. G. et al. (1991). Conducting epidemiologic research in a minority community: Methodological considerations. *Journal of Community Psychology*, 19 (1), 3–12.

Myers, V. (1979). Survey methods and socially distant respondents. *Social Work Research and Abstracts*, 15, 3–9.

Neighbors, H. W. (1983). Seeking professional help for personal problems: Black Americans' use of health and mental health services. *Community Mental Health Journal*, 21 (3), 156–171.

Neighbors, H. W. (1984). The distribution of psychiatric morbidity in black Americans: A review and suggestions for research. *Community Mental Health Journal*, 20, (3), 169–181.

Neighbors, H. W. (1987). Improving the mental health of black Americans: Lessons from the community mental health movement. *Milbank Memorial Quarterly*, 65 (Suppl. 2), 348–380.

Neighbors, H. & Jackson, J. (1986). Socioeconomic status and psychological distress in adult blacks. *American Journal of Epidemiology*, 124, 779–793.

Neighbors, H. W. & Lumpkin, S. (1990). The epidemiology of mental disorder in the black population. In D. S. Ruiz, ed., *Handbook of Mental Health and Mental Disorder Among Black Americans*. Westport, CT: Greenwood Press, 56–66.

Nolen-Hoeksema, S. (1987). Sex differences in unipolar depression: Evidence and theory. *Psychological Bulletin*, 101, 259–282.

Olmedo, E. L. & Parron, D. (1981). Mental health of minority women; Some special issues. *Professional Psychology*, 12, 103–111.

Paskin, H. A. (1929). Brief attacks of manic-depressive depressions. *Archives of Neurology*, 22, 123–134.

Paykel, E. S. (1991). Depression in women. *British Journal of Psychiatry,* 158 (suppl.10), 22–29.

Paykel, E. S. & Cooper, Z. (1991). Life events and social stress. In E. S. Paykel, ed., *Handbook of Affective Disorders,* 2nd ed. Edinburgh: Churchill Livingston.

Phillips, K. A., Gundeson, J. G., Triebwasser, J. et al. (1992). An empirical study of depressive personality disorder. Presented at the American Psychiatric Association, 145th Annual Meeting, May, *Abstracts,* 197.

Pincus, H. A. & Fine, T. (1992). The 'anatomy' of research funding of mental illness and addictive disorders. *Archives of General Psychiatry,* 49, July.

Quesada, G. M., Spears, W. & Ramos, P. (1978). Interracial depressive epidemiology in the Southwest. *Journal of Health and Social Behavior,* 19 (1), 77–85.

Radloff, L. S. (1977). The CES-D Scale: A self-report depression scale for research on the general population. *Applied Psychological Measurements,* 1, 385–401.

Robins, L. N. & Reiger, D. A. (eds.). (1991). *Psychiatric Disorder in America: The Epidemiologic Catchment Area Study.* New York: Free Press.

Romanowski, A. J., Folstein, M. F. & Nestadt, G. (1992). The epidemiology of psychiatrist-ascertained depression and DSM-III depressive disorders. Results from the Eastern Baltimore Mental Health Survey Clinical Reappraisal. *Psychological Medicine,* 22, 629–655.

Salgado de Snyder, V. N. (1987). Factors associated with acculturative stress and depressive symptomatology among married Mexican immigrant women. *Psychology of Women Quarterly,* 11, 475–488.

Shore, J. H., Manson, S. M., Bloom, J. I., Keepers, G. & Neligh, G. (1987). A pilot study of depression among American Indian patients with research diagnostic criteria. *American Indian and Alaskan Native Mental Health Research,* 1 (2), 415.

Spitzer, R. L., Endicott, J. & Robins, E. (1978). Research diagnostic criteria rationale and reliability. *Archives of General Psychiatry,* 35, 773–782.

Thomas, A. & Sillen, S. (1972). *Racism and Psychiatry.* New York: Brunner/Mazel.

Torres-Matrullo, C. (1976). Acculturation and psychopathology among Puerto Rican women in Mainland U.S. *American Journal of Othopsychiatry,* 46, 710–719.

Uhlenhuth, E. H. & Paykel, E. S. (1973). Symptom intensity and life events. *Archives of General Psychiatry,* 28, 473–477.

U.S. Bureau of the Census, Current Population Reports (1988). *Money, Income and Poverty Status in the U.S.: 1987* (Series p-607, No. 161). Washington DC: U.S. Government Printing Office.

U.S. Bureau of the Census, Population Reports (1989a). *Projections of the Population of the U.S. by Age, Sex and Race: 1988–2080* (Series p-25, No. 1018). Washington, DC: U.S. Government Printing Office.

U.S. Bureau of the Census, Current Population Reports (1989b). *Marital Status and Living Arrangements, March 1988* (Series p-20, No. 433). Washington, DC: U.S. Government Printing Office.

Ussher, Jane. (1991). *Women's Madness: Misogyny or Mental Illness.* Amherst: University of Massachusetts Press.

Wacher, H. R., Mullejans, R., Klein, K. H. et al. (1992). Identification of cases of anxiety disorders and affective disorders in the community according to

ICD-10 and DSM-III-R by using the Composite International Diagnostic Interview (CIDI). *International Journal of Methods in Psychiatric Research,* 2, 91–100.

Weissman, M. M. (1987). Advances in psychiatric epidemiology: Rates and risks for major depression. *American Journal of Public Health,* 77, 445–451.

Weissman, M. M. & Klerman, G. (1977). Sex differences in the epidemiology of depression. *Archives of General Psychiatry,* 34, 98–111.

Weissman, M. M., Myers, J. K. & Tischler, G. L. (1985). Psychiatric disorders (DSM-III) and cognitive impairment among the elderly in a U.S. urban community. *Acta Psychiatrica Scandinavica,* 71, 366–379.

Weissman, M. M. & Slahy, A. E. (1973). Oral contraceptives and psychiatric disturbances: Evidence from research. *British Journal of Psychiatry,* 123, 513–518.

Williams, D. H. (1986). The epidemiology of mental illness in Afro-Americans. *Hospital and Community Psychiatry.* 37, (1), 42–49.

Winokur, G. (1973). Depression in the menopause. *American Journal of Psychiatry,* 130, 72–93.

Wittchen, H.-W., Eassau, C. A., Von Zerssen, D. et al. (1992). Lifetime and 6-month prevalence of mental disorders in the Munich Follow-Up Study. *European Archives of Psychiatry and Clinical Neuroscience,* 241, 247–258.

Woods, N. F., Lentz, M., Mitchell, E. & Oakley, L. D. (1994). Depressed mood and self-esteem in young Asian, Black and White women. *American Health Care for Women International,* 11, 242–262.

World Health Organization. (1992). *The ICD-10 Classification of Mental and Behavioral Disorders.* Geneva: WHO.

Worthington, Cassandra. (1992). An examination of factors influencing the diagnosis and treatment of black patients in the mental health system. *Archives of Psychiatric Nursing,* 6 (3), 195–204.

PART II

SOCIAL ISSUES

8

African-American Homeless Women

Juanita K. Hunter

The primary causes of contemporary homelessness in the United States
include lack of affordable housing and poverty. This crisis should be examined in light of the economic, political, and societal forces that have
shaped the African-American experience in the United States. That experience was rooted in slavery, and although more than 300 years have
elapsed since then, African-Americans have yet to rid themselves of the
aftermath of inhuman bondage. Today, African-Americans continue to
face persistent, discriminatory, and access barriers to the many resources
that would enable complete self-actualization. On a daily basis, African-
American women face gender bias from both African-Americans and the
white majority.

BACKGROUND

Homelessness is not a new phenomenon for African-Americans and can
be traced throughout the history of man. Historically, black slaves were
often countryless, homeless, and were not recognized as persons in their
own right. From the beginning of slavery, blacks were brought to America
in bondage and concentrated in the South. The Civil War removed some of
the restrictions on their mobility. The attitudes, laws, and discriminatory

practices of the South, after the Civil War and during Reconstruction, kindled a desire and quest among many freed slaves for new ways of living and working. African-American women such as Sojourner Truth were strong leaders who spearheaded the movement to freedom. The end of the Civil War brought a considerable increase in homelessness and transiency. During that era, there was no significant social welfare "safety net" to protect individuals and families from catastrophe. The significant migration of blacks between the Civil War and World War I was from rural southern areas to cities within the South.

By the late 19th century, homelessness was institutionalized within the skid rows of American cities. Homelessness is typically associated with individuals who have utilized all available resources for income and housing, or those without a tangible support system. Few individuals elect this nomad way of life. That is why single men previously comprised the bulk of the "identified" homeless. The number of homeless persons increased until the late 1920s, when technological changes drastically reduced the demand for unskilled labor (Rossi, 1989). With the advent of the Great Depression in the 1930s, homelessness increased greatly. As had previously occurred during World War I, World War II reduced the homeless population. The permanent unemployed of the 1930s virtually disappeared during this period. After the war, the skid rows were identified as a collection of cheap hotels, restaurants, bars, employment agencies, and churches. African-Americans were generally not included in this grouping, nor were they visible, except in certain religious missions.

The great migration started in 1915 and the proportion of blacks living in the North and West increased to 23.8% by 1940 (Myrdal, 1944). The post–Civil War migration brought a steady stream of African-Americans to northern cities, and this trend increased during World War II. Throughout this period of migration, many African-Americans found themselves homeless. Others became homeless through loss of family ties, when husbands or other family members preceded them to the northern cities.

In conjunction with these phenomena, major changes were necessitated in their daily lives, as the traditional ways of earning a living, habitation, and social interaction drastically changed in urban versus the familiar rural communities. However, the experiences of slavery had fostered a kinship, and the religious basis of their subculture softened this reality for many. Urban housing patterns did not enhance the close-knit relationships to which many were accustomed, and thus the familiar extended families and kinship support systems were severed.

SCOPE OF THE PROBLEM

Homelessness has clearly taken on new dimensions in the 1990s. The distressing prediction that the problem will continue to increase in severity and scope seems destined to become a reality. Further, the majority of homeless persons in large urban areas are now African-American with increasing numbers of women (Burt & Cohen, 1989). While an accurate number of homeless persons has yet to be quantified, current estimates of the homeless range from 250,000 to some 3 to 4 million. Homeless families now comprise approximately 35 to 50% of the homeless group (Davidhizar & Frank, 1992; Jackson & McSwane, 1992; Coogan & Mason, 1992).

Of significance for African-Americans is that one in five children in the United States live in poverty, and the fastest growing subgroup within the homeless population are single women with children (Velsor-Friedrich, 1993; Interagency Council on the Homeless, 1991). The growth of female-headed households living in poverty increases the potential for homelessness (Bassuk, 1993). More than half of homeless children are under six years of age. In spite of these trends, the populations studied have been predominantly male (Skelly et al., 1990). Consequently, we know very little about homeless women and, particularly, African-American homeless women (Goering et al., 1990).

CAUSES OF HOMELESSNESS

Homelessness is a multifaceted problem that results from several primary factors, most often a loss of housing. Economic conditions, periods of war, natural disasters, and catastrophes add to the number of homeless. The situation has been precipitated by major changes in housing patterns after World War II, which included movement to the suburbs, demise of federal support for low-income housing programs, and a dramatic decrease in affordable housing in urban areas. In addition, the end of the War on Poverty and similar programs for addressing social and economic inequities decreased community support for indigent individuals (Hunter, 1995).

In today's rapidly changing society, technology, loss of unskilled jobs, lack of affordable housing, and poor education are viewed as major contributors to homelessness. In addition, the increased divorce rate, personal crises, and domestic violence create situations in which homelessness can more readily occur. These risk factors are further highlighted, given the fact that minority women and women living in poverty are at high risk for victimization by violence (Browne, 1993). Social problems such as the epidemic of teenage pregnancy, more single-parent families, and substance abuse may increase the numbers of homeless (Breakey et al. 1989; Bassuk, 1993; Wagner & Menke, 1992). Contemporary homelessness is at an all time high (Prentice, 1993) and the consequences disproportionately affect African-American women.

Now we have a situation wherein women of color are the majority recipients of services provided in homeless shelters in most large urban areas (Breakey 1989). The systemic, structural, and economic forces that create a disproportionate number of poor female-headed households must be considered in any discussion of contemporary homelessness (Bassuk, 1993). In the past, the strength of African-American women was applauded and criticized at the same time. The applause came as many of these women accepted the challenge to overcome against all odds and did so. However, this tended to create female-dominated households, which to some extent suppressed the role of African-American males and encouraged abandonment by many of them. African-American women were criticized and blamed for these negative outcomes.

With the changing structure of the African-American family and the diminishing support of the extended family, many more women are vulnerable to becoming homeless. In addition, the dramatic increase of young African males who are imprisoned, and those who die early because of violence, has dramatically decreased possibilities of marriage for many young African-American women. The pervasive racism in this country has contributed to increased numbers of homeless African-American women.

Homeless women are confronted with multiple, simultaneous crises at a time when their self-esteem and coping mechanisms are significantly diminished. Precipitating causes of their homelessness may vary from family violence, disputes with family members or landlords, evictions, or fires.

Complicating factors, such as alcohol and/or substance abuse, coupled with poor management skills, may further exacerbate women's needs and compromise their problem-solving skills. Homeless women with children present other unique challenges and situations. Regardless of the multiplicity of precipitating factors and causes, commonalities exist in the experiences of homeless women.

WOMEN ON THE STREETS

Homeless women on the streets reflect the long-term neglect of the many individuals who may have chronic mental illness, personality disorders, or disaffiliation from a home base. They may also be women who resist the admission policies and regulations of a traditional homeless shelter, or may view the streets as a safer place than a shelter (Bachrach, 1987). Still others may be on the streets as a result of eviction or rotation out of a shelter. Whatever the reason, women on the streets are more vulnerable to personal assaults and may become victims of crime and rape. The threat of violence for them is ever present. They are also at risk for health problems such as respiratory infections, skin disorders, and hypothermia in colder climates. Foot problems are rampant because many of these women walk for long distances with poor footgear. Other health problems such as varicose veins and chronic edema of the lower extremities are prevalent. These women may be resistant to accepting help from traditional health-related and social service systems, and rely primarily on the social network of individuals they develop for support.

WOMEN WITH CHILDREN

Homeless women with children represent the end result of financial, housing, and social deficits of the very poor. Family structure and cohesion are continuously burdened with the pressures and stressors related to basic survival. They have multiple crises, most notably the disruption and trauma of losing their housing. It becomes difficult to function as consistent and supportive parents in such a situation. This group exhibits high levels of anxiety, uncertainty, and chaos in their lives, as the full responsibility for the children is placed upon the homeless mother, who must parent under less-than-desirable circumstances. The lack of affordable day care options and baby-sitting services within shelters may interfere with the satisfaction derived from motherhood.

Many shelters have no child care services and thus the mother is responsible for her children over a 24-hour period. Mothers in these situations do not have an outlet for the release of tension so common for unsheltered mothers. The least deviation from perfection may spur some overzealous staff member to report the mother for child neglect or abuse. At times, the suspect behavior may simply represent cultural differences in child-rearing practices.

In a study of homeless women with children in which 66.7% of the subjects were African-Americans, 64.3% of the African-Americans reported no father figure in the family. When compared to Caucasian women, 64 African-Americans versus 30 Caucasian-American women were determined to be candidates for referral for additional psychological testing (Warren et al., 1992). Because of the multiple and simultaneous issues with which they are dealing, the mother's attention span is limited and it is difficult at times for her to provide constructive disciplinary boundaries for the children. The chaotic circumstances of their lives is often displayed in the behavior of the children (Hausman & Hammen, 1993). Acting out behavior, regression to bed wetting and other earlier behaviors, and temper tantrums are not uncommon.

WOMEN IN SHELTERS

Homeless shelters were primarily established to address food and shelter needs of single homeless men, but they have undergone major changes with the dramatic increase of homeless women and families. More family-oriented shelters are available and many of them now provide health, financial, social, and other services. However, the structure, comprehensiveness, and continuity of the services provided in the shelters often falls short of the pressing needs of the recipients. While some model programs do exist, many others have experienced difficulties with client selection, program approaches, and inappropriate staffing mixes.

In Buffalo, New York, the Nursing Center for the Homeless was a project sponsored by the School of Nursing at the State University of New York at Buffalo and funded by the Division of Nursing from 1987 to 1993 (Special Project Grants Program, 1993). The project established health and related services for women at two sites. They included health assessment, health interventions, health education, referrals, social services, and transportation. These services were specifically focused on women's issues, when it became apparent that the special health, emotional, and social needs of this group were not being addressed in more traditional settings.

Typically, homeless women clients came from low socioeconomic backgrounds and were destitute. Homeless women often arrived at the shelter after having been evicted with dependent, frightened children; fleeing an abusive partner; or other unsafe situations. Some had no coats or boots on in the middle of winter and came only with the clothes on their backs. Homeless women with mental health problems had often been shifted from one mental health facility to another, with little continuity in their care. Many had been victims of sexual and/or physical abuse. Also, those presenting with unmet health needs often demonstrated underlying emotional psychiatric problems. These women were in crisis and without power. They arrived at the clinic site unable to adequately cope with the multiple factors that caused their homelessness. Their usual and reasonable alternatives had been exhausted to address the individual, economic, and family issues that precipitated their homelessness in the first place. Their immediate needs were food, shelter, housing, and safety. African-American women now comprise more than 75% of this group.

Data from this project documented that more than half of the women were single, had a mean age of 35 years, and 63.6% had a high school diploma or GED (General Education Diploma). There was an average of two children per family. Forty-two % of the parents were single. While they were predominately "local" homeless versus those who had come from other states, they still felt isolated and alone. Their support systems were no longer functional or were nonexistent. The women often argued, were critical of each other, and became frustrated due to the lack of control over their lives (Special Project Grants Program, Final Report, D10 NU6004-04, 1993).

HEALTH PROBLEMS

The data clearly demonstrate that homeless women generally manifest some common patterns of poor health that occur repeatedly. Toothaches and caries, draining and damaged teeth are almost the norm, secondary to battering, poor oral hygiene, and last-resort dental care, which generally ends up in multiple extractions. Gynecological problems related to sexual abuse, sexually transmitted disease, and inadequate care are common. Pregnant women often do not receive prenatal care. Other often-seen problems include depression, nutritional deficiencies, infestations, alcohol and drug abuse, and social isolation, to name a few (Breakey et al., 1989; Burt & Cohen, 1989; Ugarriza & Fallon, 1994). Assessment of their health needs indicated a lack of coordinated regular medical, dental, and prenatal care (Adkins & Fields, 1992). These women were often in need of mental health services, particularly those who had been victims of domestic violence. Furthermore, data confirmed that homeless single women have higher rates of psychiatric disorders than homeless men (Buckner et al., 1993).

Of particular concern is the risk of homeless women and particularly African-American women for several potential life-threatening diseases. Startling trends recently have been reported related to the spread of HIV/ AIDS. The incidence of AIDS is increasing more rapidly among women than men. In 1993, among women aged 25–44 in the United States, AIDS was the fourth leading cause of death. More than three-fourths (77%) of cases among women occurred among blacks and Hispanics, and rates for black and Hispanic women were at least 16 times higher than those for white women (Ungvarski, 1995; CDC, 1995). The majority of children infected with HIV are born to African-American women and Latinas (Ungvarski, 1995).

Homeless women, in general, are at greater risk for infection due to engaging in prostitution and other high-risk behaviors. Many are raped, are intravenous drug users, or mentally ill. They represent a very endangered group. HIV testing may be done, yet the woman may have left the shelter before the results are given to her. In a recent survey, it was found that many women did not follow up for gynecological care because they forgot their appointments. Also, they did not want to leave the safe environment of the shelter to keep outside appointments (Johnstone et al., 1993). The upsurge of tuberculosis after many years of decline is believed to be related to the HIV epidemic. Persons who have compromised immune systems by HIV are much more susceptible to developing Tuberculosis (Colson et al., 1994).

The health status of African-Americans continues to be an issue. Historically, African-Americans were denied health care because of segregation and discrimination. An extensive folk medicine practice was utilized by many African-Americans, in part a response to the lack of access to medical and hospital care. Today, many of the access barriers have been removed. However, many African-Americans still receive less-than-adequate health care, are disproportionately cared for in hospital clinics, and have poorer health care outcomes. African-Americans continue to experience higher rates of chronic diseases, such as cancer, heart disease, and strokes,

and live an average five years less than Caucasians. As a group, they tend
to ignore symptoms until they become intolerable, and thus are more often
diagnosed when diseases have already caused permanent damage.

African-American women have higher rates of infant death, diabetes
mellitus, breast cancer, hysterectomies, and tubal ligations. While a significant number of African-American women are obese, their nutritional
status is often below average. Dietary patterns that are culturally determined contribute to this problem and are difficult to change. In addition,
African-American women, and particularly homeless women, have very
little knowledge or accurate information about their own bodies. For example, it is not unusual for some of these women to be unaware of safe
sex practices. Many freely admit to unprotected sex.

ISSUES OF PROVIDING CARE

Given the current situation of the health of African-Americans, the challenge of providing health care and appropriate follow-up for homeless
women is a major one. In general, they do not seek health care in a timely
manner. Often, other women or shelter staff must encourage the client to
go to the health clinic. This reluctance is due to several factors. First, because they have so many pressing concerns in the shelter, health care is not
an immediate priority. Second, many of these women have had negative
experiences with other health care providers, and particularly with white
male physicians. And third, most of the women do not have health insurance, and paying for care is a major barrier.

Even though services provided in the Buffalo Nursing Center were free
of charge to clients, barriers still existed. Follow-up and continuity of care
was difficult. Culture reports take a week or longer to be reported, and
results may be received after a client has left the shelter. Women in the
shelter rarely leave a forwarding address. Some give a false address, making it nearly impossible for shelter staff or the Health Department to notify
them, particularly if their diagnosis required treatment.

Generally, the women in Buffalo lacked knowledge of health maintenance and health promotion approaches (Adkins & Fields, 1992). Health
services were provided in the shelter for episodic conditions and for health
problems amenable to intervention and treatment. The women often refused to accept referrals to other clinics and hospitals, due to possible em-
barrassment about their current homeless situation, long waits, inability to
pay for services, and negative attitudes of health care professionals.

ISSUES OF POWERLESSNESS

Life in a shelter is stressful and crisis-prone. Women enter the shelter
environment dealing with a series of dramatic and traumatic events.

Within this environment they lose further control over their lives. Adult women are required to live in cramped quarters, share meals with total strangers, and face a bureaucratic system that is not always user friendly. Mandates are often imposed on them without benefit of a complete assessment of their needs. What these women need, first and foremost, is acceptance and nonjudgmental understanding. Women in the shelter often make reference to the lack of sensitivity of staff, as they are pushed to apply for social services and make contacts with housing agencies. Shelter staff may be inexperienced, nonprofessional, and lack cultural awareness. Often they have few skills and inadequate training to assist women in emotional crisis or those in need of immediate psychiatric help.

The Buffalo Nursing Center project staff assessed the situation and determined that these women needed support, information, and linkage to other community resources. For example, priority one from the agency perspective was for the resident to apply for social services. Priority two was to seek housing. While mental health, physical health, and social needs were overriding factors, they were not usually considered as immediate priorities. Far too many women did not receive help appropriate to their needs. Many relied on informal networks developed with other women in the shelter, which often resulted in receiving inaccurate or incomplete information. Likewise, if children had physical problems, they were sometimes ignored until symptoms become pronounced and unmanageable.

SUPPORT GROUP

The Nursing Center staff developed an innovative approach to easing the tensions of the women in one specific shelter. The development of a mutual support group was a response to the women's demonstrated need, and provided an outlet for release of pent-up feelings. The group was convened during evening hours on a weekly basis and baby-sitting services were provided by volunteers. Nursing staff encouraged the residents to attend prior to the scheduled meeting time. They also reassured them that the purpose of the meeting was to address their concerns and was not mandated by shelter administration. Each session was staffed by a psychiatric/mental health nurse/clinical specialist and a community health nurse. The process was open ended and each participant was encouraged to share pressing events in her life. Each session provided an opportunity for a catharsis of feelings and acknowledgment of needs/problems and concerns in a quiet, nonthreatening environment.

In most sessions, in an unthreatening environment, the women were candid, open, and brought forth concerns about safety, incest, abuse, violence, and substance abuse, to name a few of the problems. The women provided encouragement to each other. As anticipated, some women were clearly in need of psychiatric/mental health follow-up. This was provided by the psychiatric/mental health nurse/clinical specialist in individual sessions after the group meeting. Appropriate referrals were made when indicated. The beneficial results included an emphasis on sharing, providing the women with information, and assisting them to focus on assessing their own personal situations.

Nursing staff demonstrated respect, trust, and recognition of each person's worth. They were interested listeners, supported each person's strengths, encouraged the women to network with each other, and to assume meaningful roles. The women learned how to access available resources and services and to maximize their efforts in doing so. These results were compatible with those discussed in the literature related to empowerment (to enable another). The positive results of empowerment have been described as gaining a sense of control over one's life and a reduction in feelings of oppression, victimization, and paternalism (Gibson, 1991; Malin & Teasdale, 1991). The results of this intervention indicated that more attention must be given to cost-effective measures to assist this special group of women to help them to regain self-esteem, feelings of self-worth, and control over their lives. Failure to do so will encourage further and chronic homelessness.

RECOMMENDATIONS

There is a critical need for comprehensive health care for homeless women. Safe havens where women can be provided with effective, quality care are desperately needed. The homeless project in Buffalo, New York, has, on a small scale, provided quality health care services to homeless women. It has also connected women and their children with a variety of health care resources within that city.

Our work in establishing the support group indicates that many of the women's immediate needs can at least be identified and recognized in a nonthreatening, supportive environment. Women can be encouraged to provide each other with support and assistance with problem-solving around issues they all face (i.e., bureaucratic maze, accessing correct information, child care needs, etc.). For many women, leaving the shelter without a comprehensive plan or collaborative efforts of providers simply predisposes them to homelessness in the future. More residential programs and quality housing are needed to provide these women with opportunities to acquire work skills, increase self-esteem and learn parenting. Additionally, transitional housing should not be used as a substitute for permanent housing. Follow-up is needed after the women leave the shelter, to reinforce new behaviors, and to prevent homelessness in the future (Kinzel, 1993).

The work of Montgomery (1994) is supportive of these findings. She conducted a preliminary investigation of homeless women to determine how they overcame their circumstances. Most of the women had been physically or sexually abused as children. Others had been neglected or abandoned by their mothers. The respondents viewed their homelessness as a temporary disruption that occurred when they attempted to change their circumstances and move on to a better life. The personal strengths that the women identified were: a stubborn sense of pride, positive orientation, moral structure, and a clarity of focus that grew out of the first three qualities. Connection with a larger community helped these women to mobilize their strengths and rebuild their lives (Montgomery, 1994).

Those individuals who work with African-American homeless women should be oriented to the special emotional/psychosocial needs of this group. Providers should be sensitive to issues of race and how this relates to their homelessness. They also need to be sensitive to the unique position of a homeless person and the related stress that threatens an individual's sense of mastery and confidence (Baumann, 1993). The loss of self-esteem, powerlessness, and victimization among these women must be addressed in order to empower them to take control of their lives. Symptoms that suggest that the homelessness will become long-term will be manifested through individuals who are unable to set directions and long-term goals or plans for "getting on with their lives." Each of these factors must be addressed with understanding and positive, culturally relevant concern if help is to be given to these clients.

SUMMARY AND CONCLUSIONS

The homeless problem in contemporary society has been created by political, economic, and societal forces that have included drastic and severe federal funding cuts in affordable housing for low-income individuals. At the same time, the stock of affordable housing in urban areas has been reduced. There are many pathways to homelessness; most include individual, family, and economic factors. The health, social, and housing needs of the women who are homeless are great and the available services are unable to meet the identified needs. African-American women are particularly vulnerable to homelessness and its consequences. There are increased numbers who are single parents. Racial discrimination continues to exist in the housing market, in bureaucratic agency policies, and in attitudes of providers.

In spite of the increasing numbers of homeless women with children, there is no national or organized program to address the multiple issues faced by homeless women. There is no public outcry for addressing the root causes of homelessness. Current programs do not effectively address the complex and long-term problems of this group. The existing federal legislation Public Law 100-77 (Stewart B. McKinney Act of 1987) authorized funding for emergency shelters and a variety of programs. This legislation does not provide for development of low-rent housing or adequate incomes for extremely poor people. With the anticipated thrust of the mid-1990s Republican-controlled Congress to further reduce assistance for the very poor, we can only anticipate even greater numbers of homeless women and children (Weinreb & Buckner, 1993).

Policymakers and public officials should recognize the effects of homelessness on individuals and families. The psychological effects and the disruption of normal parenting are cause enough for action. Without attention, all indications are that this problem will threaten the physical and mental health of the next generation of American citizens, and particularly those who are African-American.

To date, concerted government support of programs to assist the homeless has been lacking. What is needed is a program of antipoverty policies and affordable housing. At a time when elected officials are forging ahead with a mandate to eliminate government control, a federal initiative is needed to coordinate resources and provide leadership to states to encourage a pro-active approach to a contemporary problem that will undoubtedly increase. The lack of health care to this group will present an ever-increasing public health problem for the majority society. The alternative will be an ever-increasing number of citizens, and especially children, who will not be prepared to compete in the 21st century. Effective, realistic, and coordinated efforts of all major helping, religious, and public housing agencies are urgently needed.

WORKS CITED

Adkins, C. B. & Fields, J. (1992). Health care values of homeless women and their children. *Family Community Health,* 15 (3), 20–29.

Bachrach, L. L. (1987). Homeless women: A context for health planning. *The Milbank Quarterly,* 65 (3), 371–396.

Bassuk, E. L. (1993). Social and economic hardships of homeless and other poor women. *American Journal Orthopsychiat.,* 63 (3), 340–347.

Baumann, G. L. (1993). The meaning of being homeless. *Scholarly Inquiry for Nursing Practice: An International Journal,* 7 (1), 59–70.

Breakey, W. R., Fischer, P. J., Kramer, M., Nestadt, G., Romanoski, A. J., Ross, A., Royall, R. M. & Stine, O. C. (1989). Health and mental health problems of homeless men and women in Baltimore. *JAMA,* 262 (10), 1352–1357.

Browne, A. (1993). Family violence and homelessness: The relevance of trauma histories in the lives of homeless women. *American Journal Orthopsychiat.,* 63 (3), 370–384.

Buckner, J. C., Bassuk, E. L. & Zima, B. T. (1993). Mental health issues affecting homeless women. *American Journal Orthopsychiat.,* 63 (3), 385.

Burt, M. R. & Cohen, B. E. (1989). Differences among homeless single women, women with children, and single men. *Social Problems,* 36 (5), 508–524.

Centers for Disease Control & Prevention. (1995). Update: AIDS among women—United States, 1994. *Morbidity and Mortality Weekly Report,* 44 (5), 81–84.

Colson, P., Susser, E. & Valencia, E. (1994). HIV and TB among people who are homeless and mentally ill. *Psychosocial Rehabilitation Journal,* 17 (4), 157–159.

Coogan, D. & Mason, T. H. (1992). Health screening for the homeless. *Nursing Connections,* 5 (3), 5–8.

Davidhizar, R. & Frank, B. (1992). Understanding the physical and psychosocial stressors of the child who is homeless. *Pediatric Nursing,* 18 (6), 559–562.

Gibson, C. H. (1991). A concept analysis of empowerment. *Journal of Advanced Nursing,* 16, 354–361.

Goering, P., Paduchak, D. & Durbin, J. (1990). Housing homeless women: A consumer preference study. *Housing and Community Psychiatry,* 41 (6), 790–794.

Hausman, B. & Hammen, C. (1993). Parenting in homeless families: The double crisis. *American Journal Orthopsychiat.,* 63 (3), 358–369.

Hunter, J. K. (1995). Homelessness: Nursing care for a vulnerable population. *Journal NYSNA,* 26 (1), 37–39.

Interagency Council on the Homeless. (1991). *The 1990 Annual Report of the Interagency Council on the Homeless.* Washington, DC.

Jackson, M. P. & McSwane, D. Z. (1992). Homelessness as a determinant of health. *Public Health Nursing,* 9 (3), 185–192.

Johnstone, H., Tornabene, M. & Marcinak, J. (1993). Incidence of sexually transmitted diseases and pap smear results in female homeless clients from the Chicago Outreach Project. *Health Care for Women International,* 14, 293–299.

Kinzel, D. M. (1993). Response to "The meaning of being homeless." *Scholarly Inquiry for Nursing Practice: An International Journal,* 7 (1), 71–73.

Malin, N. & Teasdale, K. (1991). Caring versus empowerment: Considerations for nursing practice. *Journal of Advanced Nursing,* 16, 657–662.

Montgomery, C. (1994). Swimming upstream: The strengths of women who survive homelessness. *Advance. Nursing. Science,* 16 (3), 34–45.

Myrdal, G. (1944). *An American Dilemma.* New York: Harper & Bros., chapt. 8.

Prentice, B. (1993). Homelessness and public policy. In J. Hunter, ed., *Nursing and Health Care for the Homeless.* Albany: State University of New York Press, 17–29.

Rossi, P. (1989). *Without Shelter.* New York: Priority Press Publications, chapt. 1.

Skelly, A. H., Kemsley, M., Hunter, J. K., Getty, C. & Shipman, J. (1990). A survey of health perceptions of the homeless. *Journal NYSNA,* 21 (2), 20–24.

Special Project Grants Program in the Nursing Education Practice Resources Branch, Division of Nursing, U.S. Department of Health and Human Services, Public Health Service, Health Resources and Services Administration, Bureau of Health Professions Administration. (1993). Grant #5D1060003-05 and Grant #2D106003-04.

Ugarriza, D. N. & Fallon, T. (1994). Nurses' attitudes toward homeless women: A barrier to change. *Nursing Outlook,* 42 (1), 26–29.

Ungvarski, P. J. (1995). HIV/AIDS Lessons learned from an epidemic. *Journal NYSNA,* 26 (1), 51–53.

Velsor-Friedrich, B. (1993). Homeless children and their families, Part 1: The changing picture. *Journal of Pediatric Nursing,* 8 (2), 122–123.

Wagner, J. D. & Menke, E. M. (1992). Case management of homeless families. *Clinical Nurse Specialist,* 6 (2), 65–71.

Warren, B. J., Menke, E. M. & Clement, J. (1992). The mental health of African-American and Caucasian-American women who are homeless. *Journal of Psychosocial Nursing and Mental Health Services,* 30 (11), 27–30.

Weinreb, L. & Buckner, J. C. (1993). Homeless families: Program responses and public policies. *American Journal Orthopsychiat.,* 63 (3), 400–409.

9

Rural Black Women's Knowledge, Attitudes, and Practices Toward Breast Cancer: A Silent Epidemic

Dolores Davis-Penn

This chapter examines the barriers that deter rural African-American women's utilization of breast cancer prevention and control programs, by providing analysis of knowledge, attitudes, and practices about breast cancer among Southeast Missouri's rural black women, and discusses culturally appropriate interventions and strategies to reduce breast cancer mortality and morbidity.

Breast cancer is the leading cause of cancer mortality among black women in the United States (Burack, 1989). Although breast cancer occurs across all races and socioeconomic classes, the incidence and mortality rates are higher, and increasing much faster, for blacks than nonblacks (Willis et al., 1989).

In 1993 it was estimated that 182,000 women were diagnosed with breast cancer. The mortality rate was extrapolated at 46,300. One out of every eight white women will develop breast cancer as compared to one out of eleven African-American women (Washington, 1995, p. 62). However, the death rate for white women increased by only .4% from 27.1 per

This chapter is dedicated to my beloved mother who died of breast cancer at the age of 49. Special thank yous are extended to Natalie Ricks, Valerie Cassell, Thomas Taku, Angel McFadden, and Andrew Erb.

100,000 in 1973 to 27.5, in 1989 while the death rate for black women increased 4%, from 26.1 per 100,000 in 1973 to 30.4 in 1989. In addition, the five-year survival rate is only 63% for black women as compared to 75% for white women (Brown et al., 1994, p. 21).

For women in their 40s, the risk of developing breast cancer is nearly the same regardless of whether they are African-American or white. The risk of death from breast cancer, however, is 50% higher for African-American women than for whites in this age group. The reasons for the higher mortality per case for African-Americans in this age group are included in National Cancer Institute Black/White Survival Study (Davis-Penn, 1993). These grim statistics underscore why African-American women are so terrified of breast cancer. As noted above, the disproportionate rise in the death rate means that although more white women get breast cancer, disproportionately more black women will die from this devastating disease.

Health programs that serve rural elderly people are often fragmented and nonresponsive to comprehensive emotional, social, cultural, and socioeconomic needs of the individual (Brown et al., 1994, p. 21). Consequently, many rural black women have developed beliefs and attitudes toward breast cancer that completely contradict prescribed medical practice. They often view a diagnosis of breast cancer as an "automatic death sentence" and adopt the attitude that the disease is a "modern day scourge" or a "punishment from God" (Davis-Penn, 1993). This fatalistic view often has a paralyzing effect by imposing a sense of powerlessness over the breast cancer victim's family, intimate friends, and neighbors. In many instances, breast cancer becomes the silent epidemic. It becomes a taboo subject, unmentionable even among close family and friends.

CULTURAL BARRIERS TO CANCER CARE

A study of rural African-American women in North Carolina with advanced breast cancer reported that after a diagnosis of cancer was received from a physician, many of the women in the study viewed cancer as a supernatural disorder that could not be treated by "ordinary means" including physician-prescribed treatments. One patient noted that "cancer is a horrible disease. It just eats you up. The only one powerful enough to overcome it is the Lord. You just have to trust in Jesus to do battle for you and save you from the horrible affliction." In this example, battle metaphor is used to portray a struggle between God as the all-powerful force for good and cancer as consummate evil or, as another woman put it, "that terrible, evil sickness."

This next example illustrates why some women will not get a mammogram even if it is free. Some believe that "If you have a lump and its not bothering you, leave it alone. You don't want to get it started. That's why

I don't hold with this idea of poking around to look for lumps. Why look for trouble? When that doctor wanted me to have the X-ray on my breast, I told him he was crazy. There's no telling what those X-rays might stir-up." The respondents also viewed cancer as a powerful and virtually un-stoppable disease once it is activated, women need to be careful "not to stir it up"; informants view cancer as a minion of fate that may punish those who notice or defy it; to think about cancer, to try to prevent it, is to tempt fate. Cancer testing is "looking for trouble." For many of the informants, even speaking the word "cancer" out loud was potentially dangerous, as was talking about the disease openly or acknowledging that others had it.

It is the belief of these rural women that refusing to name the disease or acknowledge that you have it protects you in some way from suffering the full effects. One respondent described her feelings after receiving a breast cancer diagnosis: "When he told me what it was, well I just couldn't hardly even think about it. To have that disease would be the end. So I just decided then and there that I wouldn't worry any more. That I would give it to God, and that I would never speak of it again, I trusted God to heal me and I believe he has. That's all I need to know." Once having made this decision the respondent refused surgery and abandoned radiation treatments. In subsequent interviews, she never mentioned cancer again. In a interview just before her death, she claimed that pneumonia was killing her. She had not mentioned the word "cancer" since the day that she received the diagnosis. These cultural barriers to one of our nation's major health problems emphasizes the serious nature and complexities that must be understood and considered before oncologists can establish therapeutic relationships with rural African-American women.

EARLY DETECTION TO SAVE LIVES

The good news is that black women do not have to accept these grim statistics as irreversible facts. Moreover, they do not have to accept this disease as an automatic death sentence and can actually save their lives and the lives of their loved ones by utilizing breast cancer prevention and control methods. Through the implementation of culturally sensitive intervention programs to increase rural black women's awareness, knowledge, and education about the life-saving early detection breast cancer prevention and control methods, they will be able to take aggressive actions to decrease the incidence of breast cancer mortality and fear among women residing in rural black communities. These preventive breast cancer detection programs will also have the added benefit of greatly reducing our society's economic costs and social burdens.

Early detection in controlled breast cancer research demonstration screening trials conducted since the early 1960s have conclusively demonstrated a 30 percent reduction in breast cancer mortality among women aged 50 and over. This protocol includes breast self-examination (BSE), clinical breast examination (CBE), and mammography screening (Price et al., 1992). In addition, women who are diagnosed when cancer is limited to the breast, and lesions are small, have a five-year survival rate of 90%. However, the survival rate drops to 18% if the cancer is not diagnosed until it has spread to other sites in the body (AARP, 1995).

Hillary Rodham Clinton declared that "Early Detection Is the Best Defense Against Breast Cancer" as she launched the White House's Breast Cancer Awareness Campaign at the 1995 White House Conference on Aging in Washington, D.C. In a 1993 news release, Health and Human Services Secretary Donna E. Shalala stated that early detection programs are needed to educate and encourage women to seek cancer screening services and are particularly important for women of racial and ethnic minorities, where mortality rates are disproportionately high.

Although women of all races underuse breast cancer screening procedures, several studies have found that not using these procedures is especially pronounced among minorities (U.S. DHHS, 1991). In 1987, 25% of women aged 50 and older reported having had a clinical breast examination and mammogram within the preceding two years. This figure was 27% for white women, 19% for African-American women, 18% for women aged 70 and over, 18% for Hispanic women, 16% for women with less than a high school education, and 15% for women with an annual income of less than $10,000. Only 38% of white women aged 40 and older reported having a mammogram, as compared to 18% of black women (Rimer, 1992). More recent data from several regional surveys suggest that substantial increases in mammography screening have primarily been among younger, better educated, married women from higher socioeconomic levels (U.S. Department of Health and Human Services, 1990).

Because of widespread underuse of breast cancer screening procedures, public and private organizations have issued guidelines and recommendations for women that, if followed, would lead to a reduction in the number of breast cancer deaths by the year 2000. The 1990 report, *Healthy People 2000: National Disease Prevention and Health Promotion Objectives,* included recommendations to address prevalent age-related risk factors that are vital in saving lives and reducing costly treatments for later-stage cancer. The objectives called for an increase to at least 80% of the proportion of women aged 40 and older who have ever received a clinical breast examination and a mammogram; and to at least 60% for those aged 50 and older who have received them within the preceding one to two years (U.S. DHHS, 1991).

At present, the National Cancer Institute recommends that women have annual mammograms starting at age 50. The American Cancer Society recommends mammograms every one to two years starting at age 40. The Centers for Disease Control also recommend that women have a baseline mammogram at age 40 (U.S. DHHS, 1991). However, some authorities do not believe that these recommendations are adequate for black women. Dr. Edwin Johnson, author of *Breast Cancer/Black Women* is quoted in Washington (1995) that black women should begin having mammograms at age 30, because they develop the disease five to six years earlier than white women and their breast cancers tend to be more aggressive. According to the National Cancer Institute, 37% of black women diagnosed with breast cancer are under age 50, compared with 22% of white women. Some studies have shown that breast cancer may develop differently in black women. In recognition of these differentials in age between black and white women, the National Black Medical Association recommends that black women have a baseline mammogram at age 35 (Washington, 1995, p. 62).

BARRIERS AND RISK FACTORS

Next to gender, age is the greatest risk factor for breast cancer. Two-thirds of all breast cancer cases occur in women over the age of 50. Although women age 65 and older comprise only 14% of the female population, they constitute 43% of the cases diagnosed with invasive breast cancer (U.S. DHHS, 1991).

Low socioeconomic status is also a major factor in the underutilization of breast cancer screening. It accounts for a large portion of the discrepancy between black and white women in the stage of cancer at diagnosis and in breast cancers survivor rates (Rimer, 1992). Washington (1995, p. 66) cites a 1992 study that says African-American and poor women are screened for breast cancer less frequently than more affluent women. The study also revealed that physicians do not test women who are at high risk for breast cancer any more frequently than they test women whose breast cancer risk is lower. This is particularly disturbing, since a study published a decade earlier in 1982 stated that when women were appropriately screened there was no differential in the survival rates of white and nonwhite groups (U.S. DHHS, 1991). According to the *Healthy People 2000 Report,* women eligible for mammography revealed that the two most important reasons that they did not receive a mammogram is that they did not know they needed it or that their doctor did not recommend it.

Black elderly women are particularly vulnerable and sustain the highest mortality rates from breast cancer. This may be attributed to the "quadruple jeopardy" effect (being black, female, old, and poor). For black elderly women who live in rural areas, these risk factors are further exacerbated by social variables including cost, accessibility and availability of health care providers, and lack of awareness, knowledge, education, and community involvement. However, surveys have shown that even when mammograms are free, 60% of women will not get them (U.S. DHHS, 1991).

To gain a better understanding of the lack of utilization of health care services, a survey was conducted for the Missouri Department of Health (Davis-Penn, 1992). The survey population consisted of 100 low-income black persons ranging in age from 18 to 56 plus living in rural southeastern Missouri. The responses provided an indication of the depth of the respondents' disregard and distrust of the health care system in their community. These feelings are illustrated by the following responses: "When I go to the doctor, I have the feeling I am treated less than a human being; I am afraid to go to the doctor" (female, age 25–35); "It is just terrible how they treat poor people. . . . Blacks die from a little scratch" (female, age 36–45); "I'd rather die at home and be comfortable. . . . I can't trust the medical profession anymore" (female, age 25–35); "I think the cost of medical care is very high. That's why some people avoid going to the doctor" (female, age 36–45); "I don't go to hospital because I am scared when I get sick they will put me in the hospital" (female, age 25–35); and "God takes care of me. Dr. Jesus is my Doctor" (female, age 56+).

As a result of the responses from this survey of rural blacks' perceptions about their health care, it is evident that any successful preventive health screening program in rural communities will have to take into account blacks' feelings of alienation about the mainstream public health system and the negative perceptions regarding the level of personal and social acceptance of public health care personnel. It follows that diversity training initiatives for health care providers will be necessary. Additionally there is a critical need for the employment of trained health care personnel who are from the same ethnic background as their patients.

A "scholarly review of health care [for] African Americans . . . in the 20th century" pointed out the importance of these variables on health:

Good health or its absence was the result of many variables, all interconnected and most related to economic status. Not only sanitary environment, but also nutrition, level of education, stress, the way one viewed and responded to illness, the availability and acceptability of medical care—all helped determine whether one was sick or well, lived or died. As for blacks, especially those in the South, institutionalized segregation heightened the effect of every other variable (Clarke-Tasker 1993).

The next section provides a detailed report and analysis of the National Black Leadership Initiative on Cancer Rural Intervention and Evaluation Project. This report will provide a basis for the development of strategic interventions and strategies that can be implemented in rural black communities to reduce incidence of breast cancer.

NATIONAL BLACK LEADERSHIP INITIATIVE ON CANCER RURAL INTERVENTION AND EVALUATION PROJECT

In October 1992, Lincoln University was one of five Historically Black Colleges and Universities (HBCUs) selected to participate in the National Black Leadership Initiative on Cancer Rural Intervention and Evaluation Project. (NBLIC-RIEP). The National Cancer Institute (NCI) awarded a three-year grant to the University of Maryland Eastern Shore to work in collaboration with four HBCUs (Lincoln University, Langston University, Shaw University, and Southern University) to develop and implement cancer prevention and control programs in rural black communities. The primary goals of the NBLIC-RIEP were (1) to reduce cancer incidence and mortality, and to improve survival rates of black Americans; (2) to address the barriers preventing blacks from gaining access to quality health care and referral to appropriate screening, diagnostic, and therapeutic cancer programs; and (3) to increase black Americans' community involvement and participation in NBLIC community outreach programs.

This innovative national program provided Lincoln University an ideal opportunity to carry out its mission as a land grant university. Lincoln University was founded in Jefferson City, Missouri, in 1866, after the Civil War, to provide educational opportunities and to meet the social needs of freed African-Americans. The Cooperative Extension program under the university's 1890 land grant status has continued the historic mission of the university by providing education, outreach, and community services to the most economically and socially oppressed African-American children, youth, and elderly citizens in rural southeastern Missouri.

Missouri was selected as one of the sites selected for this project because of the unusually high incidence of cancer among blacks in Missouri. According to the Missouri Department of Health, breast and cervical cancer mortality rates for black Missourians is more than three times higher than that for white Missourians. Cancer is also one of the few major causes of death that has risen over the past 35 years. In 1994, the American Cancer Society (ACS) estimated that there would be 27,500 new cancer cases in Missouri. The highest cancer rates for breast, cervical, and lung cancer are found among Missouri's largest concentration of black farmers and low-income older black women in the six "Bootheel" counties in southeastern Missouri.

The U.S. Census Bureau ranks the counties in the Bootheel region as some of the poorest in the nation's 3,141 counties. Over 25% of the population in this region live below the poverty level. This is brought about by the region's loss of industry and a continuing loss of population, except for dependent children and elderly residents, who are primarily dependent upon transfer government programs.

Thirty-five persons from rural southeastern Missouri and representatives from public and private organizations were selected to serve as advisors and direct the implementation of the NBLIC-RIEP. One of this committee's major responsibilities was to identify strategies to maximize possible participation and involvement in the NBLIC program.

The NBLIC project director also established a collaborative relationship with the director and staff of the Missouri Department of Health (MDOH), Bureau of Chronic Disease Prevention and Health Promotion (BCDPHP), Breast and Cervical Cancer Control Project (BCCCP), and the MODH Office of Minority Health (OMH). MDOH was one of over 17 state departments funded by the Centers for Disease Control (CDC) to develop and implement the congressionally mandated five-year Breast and Cervical Cancer Control Project. This collaborative endeavor between NBLIC-RIEP and BCCCP provided Lincoln University an unprecedented opportunity to use the resources of three federal agencies (NCI, CDC, and USDA), two state MDOH Divisions (BCDPHP), local health departments in the Southeastern Missouri Bootheel Region, and community health advocates to work together toward the implementation of a shared mission: to reduce the incidence of cancer among rural black women in Missouri's Bootheel communities. With its rich heritage of educating and promoting civil rights of African-American residents in the Bootheel, Lincoln University is uniquely qualified to provide a leadership role in the development of this interagency cooperative endeavor.

KNOWLEDGE, ATTITUDES, AND PRACTICES SURVEY

The Knowledge, Attitudes, and Practices (KAP) pilot survey patterned after the NCI 1983 Cancer Prevention Awareness Questionnaire Survey was administered as a part of the NBLIC-RIEP. The primary objective of the pilot survey was to gain a better understanding of rural blacks' perceptions of cancer risk, prevention, and treatment and to obtain baseline data regarding the means of delivery of culturally appropriate public education and outreach activities designed to increase cancer survival rates.

The communities in which the surveys were conducted are located in the counties of New Madrid and Pemiscot. This predominately rural farming region is approximately 200 miles southeast of the St. Louis Metropolitan area. According to a published county-by-county index, nearly 90% of the land is used for farming in the counties in which the target population resides (Pemiscot 89% and New Madrid 88%). Statistics from the University of Missouri, Office of Social Economic Data Analysis, indicated that the population for Lilbourn and Hayti Heights is 440 and 893, respectively. Lilbourn has an African-American population of approximately 16% and Hayti Heights' entire population is African-American. The poverty level is high in both communities, at approximately one in four (26.4%) and one in three (35.3%), respectively.

The target population for this study were African-Americans over age 18. The largest age group represented in this study were 31–40 years of age. Residents participating in the survey were selected by a random sample. Interviews were stationed at city halls, grocery stores, and other retail locations. The overall participation in this survey was overwhelmingly high; the majority of residents were willing to take part in it. Some even recruited other participants. This analysis is based on 48 completed interviews. Upon completion of the survey, results were entered into a statistical analysis cross-tabulation computer program. Results of the open-ended questions were analyzed manually.

Question 1: Would You Describe Your Overall Health As . . .

The majority of the individuals surveyed described their overall health as fair (39.6%), excellent (22.7%), and good (22.9%), followed by poor (2.1%) and 8.3% who said that they did not know the state of their overall health. For the purpose of this analysis, we grouped excellent and good together, and fair and poor together. Viewing the data in this manner shows that, generally, respondents perceived their overall health as "middle of the road"; approximately 45% of the respondents rated their health as excellent to good and 46% rated it as fair to poor.

Question 2: Are There Any Particular Things That You Do To Improve Your Health Or Just To Stay Healthy?

The majority of the population surveyed (66.7%) indicated that there were particular steps taken to stay healthy. The specific measures were examined in question 3 on the survey and are discussed next.

Question 3: What Things Do You Do Or Have You Done To Improve Your Health Or To Stay Healthy?

The following information is based on the positive responses of the 66.7% of the population that responded with yes to question 2. The most frequent responses are listed first and the least frequent listed last: exercise, eat a balanced diet, refrain from smoking, regular doctor's visits, adequate rest.

Question 4: Health Problems: For Each One, Tell Me Whether You Consider It To Be A Serious Health Problem. You Can Answer "Yes," "No," Or Don't Know."

The health problems mentioned were high blood pressure, cancer, stroke, herpes, diabetes, ulcers and AIDS. The analysis indicated that the majority of the respondents viewed all of these health problems as serious; 91.7% of the respondents viewed AIDS as serious.

Question 5: Tell Me Which Of Those You Consider The Most Serious, Second Most, And Third Most.

Again, not all participants were asked to respond to this question. Only the participants who responded positively to at least two health conditions in question 4 were asked to respond to this question. Health problems were ranked in the following order:

1. AIDS   66.6%
2. Cancer   43.0%
3. High blood pressure   37.0%

Question 6: I'm Going To Mention Some Health Problems And You Tell Me The Ones You Believe Are Caused By The Way We Live. Again, You Can Respond "Yes," "No," Or "Don't Know."

Based on analysis of the responses to this question, it appears that most of the respondents believe that all of the conditions mentioned (high blood pressure, stroke, herpes ulcers, AIDS) except for cancer are caused "by the way we live." An analysis of the responses relating to cancer and lifestyles indicated that respondents are not certain what causes cancer; 33.3% of the responses fell into each category "yes," "no," or "don't know." In the author's opinion, this indicates the need for education relative to the impact that one's lifestyle may have on preventing cancer.

Question 7: What Are Some Things That People Do That Are Risky To Their Health?

The following "risky behaviors" were named by the respondents, listed in descending order of frequency: smoking, drinking alcohol, bad eating habits, unprotected sex, inadequate rest or exercise, stress.

Question 8: In The Following Four Statements, I'd Like You To Tell Me Whether You "Strongly Agree," "Agree," "Disagree," Or "Strongly Disagree" With Each One.

A. People today seem more concerned about their health than ever before.
B. It seems like everything causes cancer.
C. The chances of being cured of cancer are better today than ever.
D. There is not much a person can do to prevent cancer

A simple majority (over 50%) did not respond strongly to any single statement. However, when the positive responses (strongly agree and agree) are analyzed in aggregate, it appears that a majority of participants generally agreed with all four statements. The highest percentage of participants (47.9%) agreed with statement A. Opinions were split regarding statement B: 33.3% agreed and 22.3% disagreed. This split in opinions regarding the causes of cancer supports an earlier hypothesis that many are uncertain as to what precisely causes various forms of cancer. An analysis of statements C and D indicated that 75% of the population surveyed believes that the chances of cancer being cured are better today than in previous years. They also believe that cancer can be prevented; 52% of the population surveyed agreed or strongly agreed with this statement as mentioned earlier; the shortcoming is that they don't know what causes or how to prevent certain types of cancer.

Question 9: For Each One Of The Following Questions, Tell Me Whether You Believe That It Can Increase A Person's Chances Of Getting Cancer.

The list below outlines potential cancer causing agents contained in the survey and indicates the percentage of respondents which said yes to this question. They are listed in descending order.

Item Named	Percent Yes
Tobacco	91.7
Sunshine	70.8
Alcohol	68.8
Birth control pills	62.5
X Ray	58.3
Bumps & bruises	37.5
Marijuana	33.3
Herpes	31.3
Drinking coffee	18.8
Foods that contain fiber	14.6
Talcum powder	6.3

It appears that the target population has an awareness level regarding certain types of cancer, namely skin and lung. However, a significant portion of the population believes that coffee and foods that contain fiber may be "potential cancer-causing agents"—18.8% and 14.6%, respectively.

Question 10: What Things Do You Believe A Person Can Do To
Reduce Her Chances Of Getting Cancer?

This question resulted in the following responses in descending order:
(1) refrain from smoking, (2) eat a balanced diet, (3) sun protection, (4)
regular physical examinations, (5) avoid the use of birth control pills, (6)
avoid X rays.

Question 11: What, If Anything, Have You Done To Reduce Your
Chances Of Getting Cancer?

Again, the responses are listed in descending order: (1) refrain from
smoking, (2) eat a balanced diet, (3) get regular physical examinations, (4)
sun protection, (5) exercise, (6) prayer.

Based on an analysis of responses to questions 10 and 11, apparently
the target population perceived them as essentially the same. Four of six
answers to these two questions *were* the same. In addition, the two most
frequent responses were the same (refrain from smoking, and eat a balanced diet). It appears that there is an awareness level relative to diet and
good health.

Question 12: I Am Going To List Some Possible Sources So That You
Can Tell Me Whether You Have Received Any Information From
These Sources About What You Can Do To Prevent Cancer. Here
The Responses Are "Yes" Or "No."

A majority of respondents (64.4%) indicated that they received information regarding cancer prevention from sources contained in the survey. The
remaining (35.4%) received additional information from health care professionals, books, and brochures. Television (77.1%), family members
(68.8%), and friends (66.7%) were the top three positive responses. An
intervention using television would produce optimal results. However, due
to budget constraints, word of mouth and hands-on type interventions
could be very effective. Interventions that involve the community or
churches would be ideal, because more than 60% of the respondents indicated that they rely on family and friends for their cancer-prevention information.

Question 13: Have You Heard Of The Following Groups?

Group	Percent Yes
American Cancer Society	91.7
The National Cancer Institute	50
Cancer Information Service	39.6
National Black Leadership Initiative on Cancer	<20
Williams Cancer Center	<20

Question 14: If A Doctor Told You About Ways To Reduce Your
Chances Of Getting Cancer, How Likely Would You Be To Try To
Follow His Or Her Advice?

Although a majority of the respondents said that they would try to follow their doctor's advice, nearly 2 out of 10 responded to this question
subjectively. They said it would depend on what the advice was, as to their
likelihood of trying to follow the doctor's instructions. Again it appears
that this type of response is an indication of the need for an educational
intervention in this region of Missouri. Perhaps providing the population
with basic cancer-prevention information would better equip them to understand and accept their doctors' instructions.

Question 15: Have You Ever Talked To A Doctor About Ways to
Reduce Your Chances Of Getting Cancer?

Seventy-five % of the people surveyed said they had not talked to their
doctor about their chances of getting cancer. Yet nearly 60% perceived
their chances of getting cancer were significant: 10.7% said very likely
and 47.6% said somewhat likely. Results of this question strengthen our
recommendations for educational intervention. Since the respondents are
not talking to their physicians concerning cancer, there is a need to educate
them and/or the persons with whom they are communicating most often
concerning cancer risk and prevention.

Question 16: What Do You Think Are Your Chances Of Getting
Cancer?

The responses to this question are listed below in descending order:

Likelihood of Cancer	Percentage
Somewhat likely	40
Very likely	27
Not very likely	22
No chance at all	10

As indicated in these study results, most of this population believe that
they have a significant chance of getting cancer.

DISCUSSION AND RECOMMENDATIONS

It is clear that the gross disparity between black and white breast cancer
mortality and morbidity rates has become one of our nation's most serious
health problems, and it is rapidly reaching epidemic proportions among
rural low-income black women. An assessment of the KAP and MDOH
surveys confirms the gravity of the situation among the low-income black

populations in two rural southeastern Missouri counties. The lack of awareness and knowledge, culturally appropriate information, and access to rural health services—combined with a segregated health care system and the respondents' feelings of alienation toward health care providers—produces a potentially dangerous and life-threatening situation for rural black women. To a great extent, this accounts for their delay in seeking medical attention, being diagnosed at much later stages of illness, and their likelihood of having a poor prognosis.

This situation is further aggravated by rural low-income black women's anxiety-ridden perceptions about cancer and deeply held beliefs, which are embedded in the cultural milieu that some diseases, like cancer, are to a large degree externally controlled. This may partially explain why some breast cancer campaigns, which are primarily targeted at white women, and utilize women's fears of cancer, have failed to reach rural black women. Campaigns designed for older rural black women need to emphasize positive messages that an annual mammogram can save one's life, instead of emphasizing negative messages that reinforce rural black women's fears and anxieties by sending the signal that you will die if you don't get a mammogram. Many rural black women feel that breast cancer is the worst possible human affliction, except for AIDS. They are particularly demoralized and devastated by the physical side effects of mastectomy, radiation therapy, or chemotherapy; and by social consequences of breast cancer treatment, all of which are perceived to be dehumanizing, causing negative and permanent alterations of their relationships with sexual partners, close friends, and family. As noted in the NBLIC survey, nearly 60% of the participants perceived their chances of getting cancer were significant, but only 25% had talked to their doctors about the disease. Because of gross misinformation, confusion, bewilderment, and lack of knowledge and education about the efficacy of utilizing breast cancer early detection methods, including monthly breast self-exams, clinical breast exam, and mammography, many rural older black women are needlessly setting the stage for their own funerals by increasing their chances of dying from breast cancer.

In conclusion, there are several projects developed to help breast cancer awareness among African-American women, but the task is far from being accomplished. Breast cancer has become the silent epidemic among rural black elderly women, who talk about it less than white women. All these factors combined result in less communication about breast cancer among rural elderly black women. As a result they are more likely to die from breast cancer than white rural elderly women. Successful intervention depends on quantity and quality of programs available to rural elderly black women. There can be a great proliferation of programs that teach rural elderly black women about breast cancer and how to prevent it, but without a culturally sensitive prevention strategy, they will fail.

This chapter has focused upon the development of culturally sensitive initiatives that can serve as a model for the delivery of community-based breast cancer control interventions. Federal, state, and local health providers and multidisciplinary teams from HBCUs can be persuaded to use these strategies to implement Afrocentric breast cancer awareness and early detection programs. They also can provide the leadership for other health care practitioners and educators in promoting preventive health trends and practices in the black population.

The lack of current, accurate information pertaining to the control and prevention of chronic diseases and the lack of access to culturally appropriate health care systems and/or organized community-based wellness programs for black elderly have contributed to citizens' pessimistic attitudes and perceptions regarding their health care.

WORKS CITED

AARP. (1995). *Perspectives in Health Promotion and Aging,* 10 (3).

Brown, Linda, W. & Williams, Roma D. (1994). Culturally sensitive breast cancer screening programs for older black women. *Nurse Practitioner,* 19 (3), 21–32.

Burack, Robert C. (1989). The acceptance and completion of mammography by older black women. *American Journal of Public Health,* 79, 721–726.

Clarke-Tasker, Veronica A. (1993). Cancer prevention and early detection in African-Americans. In Marily Frank-Stromborg and S. J. Olsen, eds., *Cancer Prevention in Minority Populations: Cultural Implications for Health Care Professionals.* St. Louis: Mosby.

Davis-Penn D. (1992). Health Care Survey. Lincoln University, Department of Cooperative Extension and the Association for Gerontology and Human Development in Historically Black Colleges & Universities and Minority Management Interns for Missouri Department of Health.

Davis-Penn, D. (1993). Interviews with southeastern Missouri rural black elderly women. August.

Price, J. H., Desmond, S. M., Slenker, S., Smith, D. & Stewart, P. W. (1992). Urban black woman's perceptions of breast cancer and mammography. *Journal of Community Health,* 17 (4), 191–204.

Rimer, B. K. (1992). Understanding the Acceptance of Mammography by Women. *Annual Behavior Medicine,* 14, 197–203.

U.S. Department of Health and Human Services, Public Health Service. (1991). *Healthy People 2000: National Health Promotion and Disease Prevention Objectives,* Conference Edition, September.

Washington, Harriet A. (1995). *Heart and Soul,* April, 66–77.

Willis, M., Davis, M., Cavins N., and Janiszewski, U. (1989). Interagency collaboration: Teaching breast self-examination to black women. *Oncology Nursing Forum,* 16 (2), 171–177.

10

Transracial Adoption: In the Child's Best Interest?

Barbara A. Seals Nevergold

Several years ago, Steve Martin starred in a movie comedy entitled *The Jerk*. In the opening scenes of the film, we're introduced to "the Jerk," Martin's character. He is an adolescent who's on the verge of leaving his southern rural home for the first time. Martin's family is comprised of mother, father, a large number of siblings and extended family members. Their home is small and somewhat cramped for the space to accommodate this rather large family. Yet, while they appear materially poor, the family is spiritually rich and expressive in their love for each other. Mama and Daddy are caring, nurturing parents who communicate their concerns openly to their son, especially advising him on how to confront and negotiate the new world into which he is venturing.

The Jerk (not the family's name for him), is a bumbling, inarticulate, uncoordinated, and naive young man. In contrast to the others he is an obvious misfit with his "family." The movie viewer can attribute this maladjustment not only to the Jerk's ineptness but to the fact that he appears to be out of sync with the rest of his family. In one scene he's the only one who can not "keep time" to the jazz music that family members like to listen to. However, the most obvious distinction between Martin's character and his "family" is immediately apparent from the very start of the movie, as he is white and they are black. Ultimately, this transracially adopted child finds himself, and his identity, beginning with his realization that not only does he like Glenn Miller, but he can move to the rhythm of Miller's music.

The humor of *The Jerk* is based on a premise that the adoption of a white child by a southern black family is not only implausible but absurd. And while that premise, as a basis for a movie comedy, may evoke smiles and laughter, the reality of transracial adoption has evoked serious debate, including accusations of racism, and has caused grave concern to members of minority communities whose children are adopted by majority group members. The concern includes questions about the future of those transracially adopted children who, unlike the Jerk, may never find their rhythm, and about the validity of the rationale that proposes that these adoptions are in the "best interests" of these children.

Transracial adoption is variously defined. For the purposes of this chapter, several definitions are cited, as they provide an indication of the complexity of this issue. Silverman (1993, p. 1) stated that "transracial adoption means the joining of racially different parents and children together in adoptive families. While this term is sometimes reserved for the adoption of black children by white families . . . it includes also the adoption of Native American, Asian, and Hispanic children by white families." Similarly, Bagley (1993) defined the transracially adoptive parents as usually white of European origin and the adoptive child as ethnically different, but recognized that this usually meant a child who was African-American or mixed-race/African-American.

Rosenthal et al. (1991) underscored the influence of this society's view of race by developing a definition that considers both the race of the child and that of the adoptive parents. If the child matched the race of at least one parent, the adoption was considered inracial, unless the child was biracial and the parents were both white. That is, a black parent and a white parent who adopt a biracial child do not constitute a transracial union. However, a biracial child adopted by two white parents is classified as transracial. The authors stressed that this racial distinction is justified in that "this social definition of race recognizes that even the suggestion of minority status in physical appearance defines the child as a minority" (Rosenthal et al., 1991, p. 20).

While the debate about the ethicacy of transracial adoption and issues that inform this debate are generalizable to all minority children, who can be described as meeting the above definitions, the focus of this chapter will center on African-American and African-American mixed-race children. A brief discussion of the history of transracial adoption follows. It is important to view this issue from both the historical and evolutionary perspectives that impacted the development of transracial adoption from an international to a domestic phenomenon.

HISTORY OF TRANSRACIAL ADOPTION

The motivations for initial transracial adoptions were largely grounded in the humanitarian efforts of Americans to provide homes for the orphans and displaced children of war. This is not to imply, however, that some of these early adoptions were not also the result of childless couples' desire to parent. Following the end of World War II, the first in a series of international adoptions occurred, in which foreign children were adopted in large numbers by white Americans. Between 1948 and 1962, more than 3,000 Japanese and nearly 1,000 Chinese children were reported adopted in this country (Silverman, 1993).

Similarly, following the Korean War, between 1950 and 1981 more than 38,000 Korean children were adopted by American families (Kim, Hong & Kim, 1979; Silverman, 1993). Koreans were generally alarmed by the large numbers of children being adopted by white Americans, and they responded by initiating a movement to curtail the exodus of children from the country. In 1974, legislation was passed that increased efforts to promote adoption within the country. In spite of these measures, however, white Americans continue to be able to adopt between 1,000 and 2,000 Korean children annually (Silverman, 1993).

The Vietnam War provided the next identifiable period in which Americans actively pursued the adoption of minority children. A significant factor that distinguishes these from other postwar adoptions, however, is that many of these children were the offspring of American soldiers and their Vietnamese partners. The adoption of these children was spurred by humanitarian relief efforts, not only to save the children from the ravages of war, but from the extreme discrimination they would endure from the Vietnamese, who ostracized mixed-race individuals. The end of the war and the withdrawal of American troops greatly reduced and subsequently led to the end of these adoptions (Silverman, 1993).

Central and South America have also been a source of adoptable children. Beginning in the 1950s, Hispanic children from countries such as Colombia, El Salvador, and Mexico have been placed in homes in this country in steadily increasing numbers. These adoptions have continued and result in approximately 1,000 children adopted annually by white families (Silverman, 1993).

The first group of American minority children to be transracially adopted in any significant numbers were Native Americans. In the late 1950s, the Indian Adoption Project was a program jointly proposed by the Bureau of Indian Affairs and the Child Welfare League of America, Inc. (CWLA). While intended as a program to place children inracially as well as transracially, the vast majority of the adoptions that resulted were transracial. Approximately 400 children were placed before opposition from the Native community ended the program. Opposition to the transracial placement of Native children was intensified following the publication of the results of a 1967 national survey, which revealed that of 696 Native American children adopted, 84% or 584 had been adopted by white families (Silverman, 1993). In 1978 the Indian Child Welfare Act was passed, which gave the right of jurisdiction over child welfare matters to Indian tribes. Thereafter continuation of transracial placements of Indian (Native American) children was prohibited by federal legislation (Jones & Else, 1979; Silverman, 1993).

The dawning of the 1960s ushered in a new era in which this historical experience with transracial adoption combined with several changes in American society to both facilitate and promote transracial adoptions on the home front. These international adoptions also sparked the development of a number of advocacy groups whose goal was to promote and support the adoption of children transracially. Groups such as the Council on Adoptable Children (COAC), Parents to Adopt Minority Youngsters (PAMY), and the Open Door Society were formed in the late 1950s and early 1960s by individuals who had adopted transracially.

These groups' goals were and continue to be the active advocacy for changes in adoption policies and legislation that will make the adoption of black and other minority children by white families easier, to provide support and education for families who have adopted transracially, and to promote transracial adoption (Ladner, 1977; Kim, Hong & Kim, 1979; McRoy & Zurcher, 1983; Rosenthal et al., 1991; Silverman, 1993). One of the responses to these efforts resulted in a revision by the Child Welfare League of America of its 1968 edition of *Standards for Adoptive Practice*. The *Standards* stated that "racial background in itself should not determine the selection of a home for a child" (CWLA, 1968).

To some degree, the Civil Rights Movement of the 1960s is credited with creating both the climate that further bolstered the goals of these advocacy groups and that which contributed to the insistent and impassioned opposition to transracial adoption (Ladner, 1977; Pohl & Harris, 1992). For many, the Civil Rights Movement was imbued with the ideals that would ultimately result in the achievement of a truly integrated society. Together, blacks and whites staged many of the offensive tactics designed to achieve equity for blacks and racial harmony in this country. Many believed that American society could eventually become one in which race would be eliminated as a barrier in human relationships.

Ladner (1977) noted that this was also a period during which a spotlight was focused on the social needs of black Americans, particularly black children. The foster care system was a special cause for concern, in that a disproportionate number of black and other minority youngsters were placed in the system. It was widely acknowledged that the system was in crisis. Foster care as a temporary measure was decried to be a hopeless failure. Children were allowed to languish or be lost in the system with little or no efforts made to reunite them with their biological families (Spar, 1991).

ACCEPTANCE OF TRANSRACIAL ADOPTION

This failure of the foster care system and the resultant lack of permanency for children was often cited as a primary impetus to justify transracial adoption. Child psychologists have identified and confirmed the psychological harm that occurs when children grow up without permanent parents. Only a few months of separation can have devastating effects on a child's development (Helwig & Ruthven, 1990; Silverman, 1993). The argument that children suffered more psychological harm from the deprivation of a permanent home than from placement in a racially different home was subsequently used for justification as adoption agencies began to reevaluate their policies on transracial adoption of black children.

Yet other changes in our society at that time provided additional mitigating factors in the movement toward transracial adoption of African-American children. Changes in birth control policies gave women the opportunity and the means to prevent unintended pregnancies and unwanted births. The decline in the number of white, adoptable babies and the correspondent large number of black children in foster care and available for adoption contributed to an environment conducive to the placement of black children with white families (Grow & Shapiro, 1974; Ladner, 1977; McRoy & Zurcher, 1983).

Modifications in attitudes about the adoption process itself were also undergoing change. Kim, Hong, and Kim (1979) noted that the previous emphasis upon finding the "perfect infant"—who closely matched the physical characteristics, ethnic background, skin color, and intellectual potential of the adoptive parents—became less relevant. The decrease in supply of healthy white infants shifted the emphasis to finding the "perfect adoptive home." This meant that the ideal adoptive parents were almost exclusively white couples, legally married, devout, respected in the community, and prosperous but childless.

The scenario was thus set for the acceptance of transracial placements of black children. The declining numbers of white adoptable children, the large number of black children available for adoption, advocacy by pro-transracial adoption groups, and the changing attitudes toward black/white relationships were the ingredients that fostered change. Adoption agencies began to actively recruit homes for these children.

Media campaigns that used television and other high visibility recruitment strategies were launched to recruit families. A major criticism of these and other recruitment methods was that they were designed for and by whites. Many of the children who were mixed African-American and white were described by terminology that would highlight their white ethnicity. As McRoy and Zurcher (1983, p. 7) state, "Such terms as 'black-white child,' 'child of mixed parentage,' 'inter-racial child,' 'part-white,' and 'bi-racial child' became common and were given positive connotation in an attempt to influence white families to consider adopting a racially mixed black child. The half-white heritage was emphasized so that white families could in some way identify racially with the adopted child."

By 1971, one-third of all black children being adopted were placed with white families (Pohl & Harris, 1992). Rosenthal et al. (1991) and others placed the number of actual adoptions that year at 2,500. Silverman (1993) estimated that between 1960 and 1977 a total of 12,000 adoptions of black children by white parents occurred.

OPPOSITION TO TRANSRACIAL ADOPTION

The first notable opposition to transracial adoption surfaced in 1972. The National Association of Black Social Workers (NABSW) approved a position paper that opposed transracial adoption. The statement, in response to issues raised by black social workers, questioned whether black children raised by whites could (1) develop positive identities, (2) learn survival skills necessary in a racist society, and (3) develop the cultural linguistic attributes crucial to function effectively in the black community (Jones & Else, 1979).

The NABSW (1972) resolution stated:

Black children should be placed only with black families whether in foster care or adoption. Black children belong physically, psychologically and culturally in black families in order that they receive the total sense of themselves and develop a sound projection of their future. . . . Black children in white homes are cut off from the healthy development of themselves as black people. . . . We have committed ourselves to go back to our communities and work to end this particular form of genocide.

Chestang (1972, p. 103), another vocal opponent, posed the question: "Can white parents equip a black child for the inevitable assaults on his personality from a society that considers his color to be enough reason to reject him? . . . How can the black child learn the necessary maneuvering, seduction, self-enhancement through redefinition and many other tactics taught by black parents, by work and deed, directly and indirectly?" Jones and Else (1979, p. 379) asserted that "the socialization of a minority child is complex because the child must be able to live and operate effectively in both the minority and majority community." Joining the NABSW and critics like Chestang and Jones and Else were other minority groups such as the Native American and black nationalist groups who saw the

Civil Rights Movement as an opportunity for these people to promote and preserve their own cultures rather than to integrate.

Although the charge of genocide by the NABSW provoked an emotional reaction from whites, it conveyed the strong belief that at a time when black people were stressing the value of their cultural heritage, transracial adoptions were a means to undermine the black community. Jones and Else argued that transracial adoption could "be viewed in large part as an expression of racism" (p. 374). They cited the adoption of the "less objectionable" minorities first, before blacks, the emphasis placed on biracial children for their lighter skin and more caucasoid features, and the failure of adoption agencies to recruit black families as rationale for their assertions.

Jones and Else assigned much of the blame for the increase in transracial adoptions to adoption agencies who not only failed to recruit black families but were inherently set up to pose systematic barriers to blacks seeking to adopt. The agency barriers to black adoption resulted from attitudes that underestimated the potential for finding homes in the black community, a bias in favor of homes in the white community, lack of knowledge of culturally relevant outreach activities, utilization of a white concept of the requirements for a good life, and lack of experience recruiting black families (Simon & Alstein 1977; Jones & Else 1979). Pointing to the fallacy of many of these issues, Pohl & Harris (1992) dispelled the myth that blacks don't volunteer to be foster parents or adoptive parents. Pohl and Harris noted that in actuality "they do so in greater numbers than other groups. Proportionately, more black people than white people give homes to children who are not their biological children" (p. 47).

Additional factors that contributed to the failure of these agencies to recruit black families is reflected in the staffing patterns, policies, and practices of these agencies. Rosenthal et al. (1991) found that approximately 838 of the caseworkers were white, and noted the lack of cultural sensitivity and knowledge of cultural differences by these staff. Minority families often found the adoption application process intimidating. Rosenthal et al. cited three studies that revealed low adoption approval rates for minority applicants. The authors surmised that these findings were probably attributable to the low educational level, income, and single-parent status of the applicants. An inherent reality that accounted for all of these barriers is reflected in the basic lack of knowledge about black culture and institutional racism and discrimination in the adoption system.

Following the mounting and vocal opposition from blacks and other minorities, many adoption agencies began to reexamine and reevaluate their policies regarding transracial placements. For a time, immediately following this initial furor, transracial adoptions of black children declined significantly. Silverman (1993) cited black-white placements in 1976 at 1,076, and an estimated 1,169 in 1987. To date, however, the exact number of transracial adoptions, or adoptions in general, can not be determined because official records have not been available since 1975 (Rosenthal et al., 1991; Silverman, 1993).

Throughout the period of this ongoing controversy, the Child Welfare League of America, the arbiter of child welfare public policy and practice, has vacillated in its support of transracial adoption. The fact that CWLA's *Standards for Adoptive Practice* have been revised several times is an indication of the difficulty that leaders within the adoption field have when confronting this issue. The 1973 edition of the *Standards* stated: "In today's climate, children placed in adoptive families with similar racial characteristics can become more easily integrated into the average family and community" (CWLA, 1973). A 1978 revision did not support the end to transracial placements but recognized the need to place a priority on same race placements. "Adoptive parents selected for a child should ordinarily be of a similar racial background, but children should not have adoption denied or significantly delayed when adoptive parents of other races are available" (CWLA, 1978).

Finally, the current revision states: "Children in need of adoption have a right to be placed into a family that reflects their ethnicity or race. Children should not have their adoption denied or significantly delayed, however, when adoptive parents of other ethnic or racial groups are available" (CWLA 1988). This position underscores the importance of the shift to a philosophy that utilizes the "child's best interest" as the basis for most foster care and adoption policy and practice decisions. The *Standards* further propose: "In any adoption plan, however, the best interests of the child should be paramount. If aggressive, ongoing recruitment efforts are unsuccessful in finding families of the same ethnicity or culture, other families should be considered (CWLA, 1988).

Even proponents of transracial adoption cited the need to maintain a connection between the child and his or her racial identity. The North American Council on Adoptable Children stressed that "transracial adopters must realize that the ethnic and cultural heritage of the child is an essential right; therefore the families must be willing to seek out services and personal contacts in the community that will support the child's ethnicity" (Hayes, 1993, p. 303).

STUDIES ON TRANSRACIAL ADOPTION

The arguments of advocacy groups, adoption professionals, social workers, and African-American and other minority-group opponents were based primarily on experiential and anecdotal evidence. A number of studies have been conducted in an attempt to establish an empirical basis for the arguments of both proponents and opponents of transracial adoption.

Throughout the literature on transracial adoption, two recurrent themes are prevalent as reflected in the research goals. First, in order to demonstrate that transracial adoption is an effective and valid alternative to inracial adoption of black children, most studies proposed designs to assess the overall adjustment of the child to his or her adoptive placement. Johnson, Shireman and Watson (1987) noted that early studies focused on characteristics of the transracial adoptive families and the child's adjustment and integration into the adoptive family. Specifically, the demographic profiles and motivations of the adoptive families, parental attitudes, and concerns about racial identity issues have been the subject of most of these studies.

Evaluation strategies to determine the child's adjustment to and integration into the family, as well as adjustment related to issues of behavior and school achievement, are often part of the design. Self-esteem assessment and measurement of the adoptive parents' and siblings' satisfaction with the adoption were also administered.

The second issue that has received significant attention in the research has been the assessment of perceptions of racial awareness and racial identity development of the black children and the impact made by the adoptive parents on that development. These studies were primarily conducted during the period between the early 1970s and mid-1980s. The following review provides a sampling of the significant studies, their findings and conclusions.

Grow and Shapiro (1974) conducted one of the earliest studies. They recruited 125 families who had adopted black children transracially. At the time of the study the children were at least six years old and had been in placement for at least three years. Interviews and questionnaires were given to the parents, while the children were given the California Test of Personality. The children's teachers, as well as the interviewers, also completed a questionnaire. The researchers compiled the results from various measures of adjustment, symptoms, adult evaluations, parental satisfaction, peer relationships, and child's attitudes toward race.

In an analysis of the data, Grow and Shapiro concluded that 77% of the adoptions were successful. These results compared favorably to the level of success found by other adoption studies for "both traditional white inracial infant adoptions and nontraditional adoptions involving racial mixtures and older children" (p. 103). In half of the 23% that were determined to be unsuccessful, the authors attributed factors such as health problems, physical and intellectual handicaps, and family catastrophes—not racial identity—for the problems. In the other half, 16 cases, the authors concluded there was evidence of conflict for the child regarding racial identity or by parents who ignored or minimized the importance of race.

McRoy and Zurcher (1983) compared 30 white and 30 black families who had adopted black children transracially and inracially. This study was significant in that it was one of the few that studied transracial adoptees who were adolescents. At the time of this study, the children were at least 10 years old and had been in the home for at least a year. The mean age of the transracial group was 13.5 years and 14.1 years for the inracial group. Symbolic Interaction Theory was used as the theoretical basis for this study. This theory "assumes a person's self-definition develops from interpersonal relations in a social world" (p. 15). And that "major influences on the development of self-concept are (1) communication directly from other people about self, (2) comparison of self with others in the immediate environment, (3) the roles assigned to self by the community" (p. 16).

McRoy and Zurcher interviewed the parents and the children separately, administered the Family Adaptability and Cohesiveness Scale to parents and the Tennessee Self-Concept Scale and the 20 Statement Test (Who Am I?) to the children. Both groups of children appeared to develop strong bonds with their parents. The parents described themselves as enjoying their children and considered the decision to adopt as a good one.

Both groups of children showed no difference on self-concept or self-esteem. On the racial identity measures, however, 56% (17) of transracial adoptees identified themselves as "either mixed, part white, black-white, human or American; 30% (9) referred to themselves as black; 10% (3) stated that their racial background was white, and one, Mexican" (p. 127). The comparison group all referred to themselves as black.

As with many of the subjects in other studies, the transracially adopted children attended predominately white schools, had little encounter with black peers, teachers, or role models. Racial differences were rarely discussed at home and the children indicated they had little or nothing in common with blacks. Furthermore, they had no desire to associate with them. The authors found that 60% of transracial parents seemed to take a color-blind attitude to racial differences. They concluded that "the parents' attitudes and their consequent actions in the selection of home and school environments have a direct relationship to the adoptees' racial self-feelings" (p. 133).

The interview data suggested a positive relationship between the adoptees self-perceptions and the parents' perceptions of the child's conception of his or her racial background. Parents who indicated human identity had children who were reluctant to focus on racial identity or identify as black. Parents who referred to children as mixed or part white had children who self-referred as mixed/part white and/or dismissed the importance of racial identity.

McRoy and Zurcher postulated that the key factor in a child's development of a positive black identity was daily contact with blacks and a corresponding positive feeling about blacks. A majority of the transracial adoptees were socialized in white communities and acculturated. Many of the transracial adoptive parents exhibited stereotypical role expectations and perceptions of blacks. The adoptees internalized their parents' views. The authors saw white parents as not responding to the necessity of equipping the child to become bicultural and to realistically perceive the historical and cultural black-white relations in American society" (p. 140).

McRoy and Zurcher's findings were not solely limited to black transracial adoptees. Studies with other ethnic groups have produced similar results. Andujo (1988) found that transracially adopted Mexican-American adolescents were more likely to identify themselves as American rather than Mexican. D. S. Kim (1977) also concluded that adolescent Korean adoptees had little sense of Korean identity and were often rejecting of the characteristically Asian aspects of their physical appearance. Of the 15 Caucasian adoptive couples in Kim, Hong & Kim's (1979) study, 10 anticipated future social difficulties for their children—for example, rejection in dating and opposition by parents of prospective daters. The remaining five did not see race as a problem.

In a series of articles Shireman, Johnson, and Watson (1986, 1987, 1988) reported outcome results of a 13-year longitudinal study on the transracial placements of 118 children. All of the children were placed at age 2 or less. The study utilized two comparison groups. The authors recruited single black parents (31), black couples (45), and white couples (42) who had all adopted black children. Parents and children were interviewed in follow-up studies at four-year intervals, when the children were 4, 8, and 13 years of age. The authors also used objective measures of intelligence, identity, and social adjustment. By 1988 attrition reduced the numbers of participants to 50 (single, 12, black, 17, white, 21).

Shireman and Johnson (1986) noted that the analysis of their earlier studies among preschool children found that the children, in all three groups, appeared to develop a positive self-concept of blackness. However, they asserted that there was some evidence that this concept may not be sustained. The first follow-up study confirmed that the positive black identity and awareness of the children in transracial homes remained constant as determined by objective measures at age 8. The researchers found, however, that the comparison group's sense of black identity intensified between ages 4 and 8.

In general, the children demonstrated a positive overall adjustment. The authors voiced concerns, however, about the ability of the parents to help the children develop and maintain black racial identity. Referring to early results, they were cautious in their interpretation. "Thus, it is apparent that the transracially adopted children are maintaining their early good sense of racial identity, but this identity is not intensifying as is that of the children in black homes. Whether this is due to the impact of parents, schools, or neighborhoods is unknown" (Shireman & Johnson 1986, p. 176). Black children had intellectual knowledge of their cultural heritage.

The authors also noted that white parents' attitudes to children's en-

counters with racial slurs and discrimination was to minimize and to react
to it as they would to general name-calling. They also minimized the importance of race, wished the child to identify with the human race, or in
some manner other than black.

A typical profile of the white families in the study described parents
with high education and occupational status. The majority lived in predominantly white neighborhoods and associated with predominantly
white friends. While the parents were aware of the need for greater contact
with blacks, most could not make the commitment of altering lifestyles.

Johnson, Shireman and Watson (1987) again raised the question of
white families' ability to establish and sustain the black identity of their
children. "The parental need to minimize the importance of race and
downplay incidents of overt racial slurs or discrimination may reflect a
family's idealism, but it may also indicate the wish to deny the child's
blackness and the value of that blackness" (p. 54). They further stated
that since assimilation of an adopted child into the family is a goal, "it is
important that the assimilation be based on the acknowledgement, not the
rejection of differences. Recognizing, understanding, accepting, and learning to cope with racial differences seem critical tasks for the child adopted
by racially different parents" (p. 54).

When the children were 13, the third follow-up study was completed.
The authors reported on school performance, self-esteem and racial identity. Parents reported serious academic and behavioral problems in 33%
of the transracial group as compared to 21% in the inracial group. The
authors concluded, however, that most of these differences were the result
of a disproportionate number of learning difficulties exhibited by the boys
in the transracial group. The age of placement was also cited as a crucial
determinant of the adjustment of the child rather than the type of adoptive
placement. The Piers Harris Self-Esteem Scale showed no differences in
self-esteem for the three groups.

Racial identity and racial performance were measured in the adolescents
by two objective tests, the Semantic Differential Test and the Social Distance Inventory, and by analyzing specific statements in interviews. Overall
assessments of racial identity as perceived by the interviewers and the parents were also incorporated. At age 8, 73% of the transracial group identified themselves as black. At age 13, all the children did. Racial preference
mean scores also did not differ significantly from the other groups. On
Social Distance, children from the transracial group were more at ease
with both blacks and whites than the other two groups. Shireman (1988,
p. 27) concluded that various measures seem to give some assurance that
these transracial adopted adolescents have developed pride in being black
and are comfortable in interaction with both blacks and whites.

Simon and Alstein (1977, 1981, 1987) conducted a longitudinal study
over a 12-year period beginning in 1972. They had 204 families who had

adopted. Of the 366 children in these families, 157 were transracially adopted. Of these children, 76% were black and the remaining 24% were Native American, Asian, or Mexican. The researchers used two comparison groups comprised of 167 biological children of the adoptive parents and 42 white adopted children. The studies were conducted in 1972, 1979, and 1984. Eighty % of the minority children were under two years at time of adoption.

The study was initiated in 1972 when the children were between 3 and 8 years of age. Information was collected through extensive separate interviews with the parents and children. The authors stated that the major purpose of the study was to explore the racial identity, awareness, and attitudes of the adopted and nonadopted children as well as perceptions, attitudes, and expectations of the families (Simon & Alstein, 1977).

In the follow-up study conducted in 1979, 71% (143) of the original families were located. At this time only the parents were involved. They were asked to complete a comprehensive questionnaire that was mailed to them. Of the 143 families, 133 completed the questionnaire, which focused on their relationship with the adopted children and birth children, on the children's relations with each other, and on what they perceived to be their children's racial identity. They were also asked questions on relationships with extended family and descriptions of their community and the children's schools (Simon & Alstein, 1981).

The 1984 study included both parents and children. The study design of the original study was utilized again. Of the original group, 96 families were interviewed. By this time the majority of the children were adolescents or young adults. Of the transracially adopted group, 111 children remained in the study; 80% were black, and the other 20% were Asian and Native American. Of particular interest to the authors was information from the transracial adoptees "about their sense of belonging in the family, the siblings' ties to each other, how they described themselves racially and socially, their scholastic and career goals, and, most of all, their feelings about having been transracially adopted" (Simon & Alstein, 1987, p. 5).

On issues of family integration and school achievement, the authors concluded that the transracial adoptees were well-integrated into their families, and that there appeared to be no significant academic or behavioral problems. They noted, however, that "as the adoptees reached adolescence, one out of every five families had profound difficulties which the parents attributed as directly related to the transracial adoption" (p. 18). On self-esteem measures, there were no significant differences in the self-concept of transracial adoptees and biological children.

Regarding the issue of racial identity and preferences, the authors found that 66% of the black transracial adoptees stated that they were proud to be black, 11% preferred to be white, and 23% said they were either mixed or did not care what color they were. About one-third of the adoptees stated that they were embarrassed when they had to introduce their parents to new friends or when they were the only nonwhite in a group. The analysis of these questionnaires revealed a remarkable finding. The authors noted that the open responses of the transracially adopting families were almost devoid of any comments on race or ethnicity. They attributed these results to the parents' utilization of denial, lack of awareness of racial issues, or reticence in addressing these issues with their children.

When asked their choice of friends, 73% of the black transracial adoptees stated they preferred "white" friends; 60% dated whites exclusively, 11% dated blacks, and 27% dated both. The authors concluded that the predominance of these preferences in dating and friendships correlated to the influence of the environment. A high proportion of the transracial adoptees lived in predominantly white neighborhoods and attended predominantly white schools.

Silverman (1993, p. 109) denoted the shortcomings of many of these studies, particularly in regard to the assessment of racial identity. In particular, he noted the difficulty of looking at this issue with adolescents and young adults. "This is not an easy task because many studies differ considerably in size, derivation, and composition of the study sample; age at placement of the adoptees; techniques employed for measuring outcome (for example, questionnaires, interviews, objective tests); age of adoptees at time of study; and the size and composition of a comparison group of adolescents, if any."

Hayes (1993, p. 303) is also critical of the validity of these studies. He observed that most of the studies measured the well-being of the adopted child and found, for the most part, that children were happy and successfully incorporated into their families and communities. However, he questioned the research on the basis that "research efforts to measure identity and heritage often appear naive. They may be based on the perceptions of Caucasian parents or simple tests that do not get at the richness and complexity of a sense of identity or knowledge of heritage."

The research appears to confirm the validity of the argument that transracial adoption offers a positive alternative to long-term foster care or institutionalization for black and other minority children. That is, the transracially adopted children were as well-adjusted, overall, as their intracially adopted counterparts. The body of research has consistently found that the majority of African-American and other minority transracially adopted children appear to adjust positively to and bond with their white families and communities. There has also been evidence that the children develop positive self-concepts.

As discussed previously in this chapter, there is substantial evidence that attests to the psychological damage to the child who is not raised in a stable environment. "Child psychologists recognize that children need the security of a loving and permanent home. Without a family to cherish them . . . they may conclude that no one wants to keep them because they are worthless (Pohl & Harris, 1992, p. 60). Since the child welfare reform movement of the 1980s, the philosophy of permanency has been the cornerstone of child welfare policy and practice. This philosophy acknowledges that a permanent family provides the child with a sense of belonging, a respected social status, and a set of relationships. Consequently, the child thrives better in a home that is permanent. The conclusions suggested by the research on transracial adoption support the assertion that there is a positive correlation between permanency and adjustment of children in transracial placements.

The research findings related to the issue of racial identity, however, have produced more debatable outcomes. It is arguable that the conclusions that can be drawn from the research strengthen the position taken by opponents to transracial adoption. Repeatedly, research results concerning the attitudes and behaviors of white parents in supporting the racial identity development of their black children illustrated the difficulty that most had in addressing this issue. While many parents acknowledged the need and attempted to expose the children to their cultural heritage, many were unable to make the commitment to sustain this exposure. Most found it equally difficult to make changes in their own lifestyles to ensure that the children had consistent and meaningful contact with black cultural influences.

For example, a significant number of parents (60% in the McRoy & Zurcher [1983] study) maintained what Ladner (1977) described as a "color blind" attitude. They preferred to stress the child's identification with the human race, or as American, mixed, or biracial. This color blindness was demonstrated in other ways by the adoptive parents. Johnson, Shireman and Watson (1987) reported that white parents' responses to their children's encounters with racial slurs and discrimination was to minimize these incidents. Essentially, they reacted to these situations as they would to general name calling. Ladner (1977) foresaw problems for adoptive parents who insisted on maintaining a color-blind attitude. She believed that this behavior would make it difficult to prepare their children for the racism inherent in American society. "Racism is a reality of society, and therefore for minorities a positive racial identity is crucial to a good self-concept. A minority child should have a clear image of himself/herself as a minority person" (p. 111).

Further evidence that white adoptive parents' ability to foster black identity development should be a concern is substantiated in the research results related to the children's attitudes and behaviors. Almost 60% of the adolescents in McRoy and Zurcher's (1983) study did not identify themselves as black. The authors concluded that a significant percentage of these adoptees were uncertain about their identity. Notably, the authors found that the adolescents' self-identity was significantly influenced by their parent's views. In most cases, they defined themselves by the same "color-blind" definitions used by their parents.

Furthermore, these teens expressed negative views of blacks and black cultural symbols. Simon and Alstein (1987) found that 20% of the adolescents in their study had adjustment difficulties that were related to their transracial adoption. Johnson, Shireman, and Watson (1987) doubted that even children whose parents exposed them to culturally relevant experiences, at an early age, could sustain a sense of racial identity over a prolonged period.

Many researchers questioned the impact of little or no daily contact with black peers and role models on the racial identity development of these youngsters. Certainly, the predominantly white communities and schools in which the majority of adoptees were raised provided a contributing factor that accounted for that lack of contact. Johnson et al. (1987) noted that assimilation is the ultimate goal of adoption. Assimilation is the end stage in the process of acculturation. The acculturated individual can be described as "having given up most of the cultural traits of the culture of origin and assumed the traits of the dominant culture" (Locke, 1992, p. 6).

The findings of these and other studies on transracial adoption confirm the belief that many transracially adopted children are acculturated. This acculturation is promoted by the attitudes and behaviors of the adoptive parents and further supported by the predominantly white environments in which they live. The result is not only the assimilation of these children into their new families, but their assimilation into the racial identities of those families as well. Consequently, many of these children adapt and assimilate, developing and identifying as white.

While numerous studies on transracial adoption have consistently documented the validity of the questions originally posed by the NABSW—that is, whether transracially adopted children would develop positive identities, learn survival skills necessary in a racist society, or develop requisite cultural linguistic attributes—these findings are usually minimized. Instead, the failure to find definitive outcomes related to the identity issue or the finding of a measure of overall adjustment are emphasized and used to justify the continued practice.

TRANSRACIAL ADOPTION ISSUES IN THE 1990S

Almost 30 years after the initial opposition to transracial adoption, the debate may again reach the level of intensity of the 1970s. Two issues are central to this debate. First, the foster care and adoption systems are populated by a disproportionate number of black, Hispanic, and other minority children. Second, the system has many of the same prerequisites that contributed to the promotion of transracial adoption as a solution to its problems. Simultaneously, traditional advocates of transracial adoption have continued to press their cause on the judiciary and legislative fronts. Several court cases have been instituted to challenge opposition to transracial adoption. In many of these cases, the courts have upheld the argument that race could not be the most important consideration in adoption (Pohl & Harris, 1992). In October 1994, President Clinton signed the Multiethnic Placement Act. "It is designed to prevent discrimination in the placement of children in foster care and adoption on the basis of race, color, or national origin. The Act prohibits states or agencies that receive Federal funds from delaying or denying the placement of any child solely on the basis of race, color or national origin" *CWLA, 1995)*.

In spite of revolutionary reform in the 1980s, the child welfare system has continued to be hampered by an ongoing crisis precipitated by many of the same problems as those of the 1960s. In 1991, after ten years of reform, the system's crisis reached monumental proportions (Pohl & Harris, 1992). Similarly, as in the 1960s, the active promotion of transracial adoption, as one response to this crisis, has again raised concern in the African-American community.

The magnitude of societal problems, for which there are no ready solutions, is compounding the crisis. At the top of the list of problems is homelessness and poverty. Over 40% of the children in care come from families on Aid to Families with Dependent Children (AFDC). Drugs and other health ailments, the most conspicuous being HIV/AIDS, contribute almost unsurmountable problems. In addition to these issues, the rapid increase in single-parent families, teen parents, two-parent working families, isolated nuclear families, and individuals with nontraditional lifestyles pose added stress on the system. The system is seriously impacted by a rapid increase in the number of children entering the foster care system, and a larger proportion of children who have significant psychological or physical difficulties. A complicating factor of this entire problem is the difficulty of recruiting sufficient foster homes.

Between 1982 and 1986, nationwide, there were approximately 286,000 children in foster care. In 1987 that number increased to 300,000, in 1988 to 330,000, and in 1989 to 360,000 (Spar, 1991). By 1991 there were more than 407,000 children in foster care (Pohl & Harris, 1992). In comparison, a 1989 CWLA study found that approximately 36,000 children are awaiting adoption (Pohl & Harris, 1992). Some 51% of these children were identified as minority. The child welfare crisis is exacerbated by the system's inability to address the needs of these children in a timely, coordinated, and systematic fashion. Barriers include systemwide inattention to adoption; changes in the makeup of the adoptable child, who is older and with special needs; and a family court that is overtaxed and moves slowly in both terminating and finalizing adoptions.

Complementing this environment is a society that, unlike the Civil Rights era of the 1960s, has moved toward an era of pluralism. Furthermore, this movement is spearheaded by minority groups who have demanded inclusiveness in American society and respect for their unique identities, histories, and achievements. The great "melting pot" society has been rejected. The values articulated by multiculturalism and diversity have provided the underpinning of this movement. In this context, transracial adoption must once again be considered in light of the arguments of the NABSW and others. This requires that the role played by the family in racial identity development is emphasized, that alternative solutions to transracial placements are sought, and that the child welfare system address and commit resources to eliminate barriers to minority participation.

Psychologists have documented the important role that families play in the socialization of children into their culture. Milner (1983, p. 53) observed that "learning the business of living in a culture is not only a question of learning skills but also of learning meanings." The foundation of learning is laid by the parents who utilize their own construction of the world, of reality. Parents thus define the child's world, explain it, and delineate its limits. Parents, consequently, are both the instructors and the interpreters of their children's societal lessons (Milner, 1983).

McAdoo (1993) emphasized the crucial role of the family in the socialization of the child as a member of his or her ethnic group. In particular, she stressed that "our ethnicity cannot be separated from our families" (p. 3). The family is the mediator of many of the ethnic culture attributes. McAdoo stated that development of positive ethnic group identity is a result of both self-perceptions and perceptions held by others outside the group. It is more difficult to raise children to have pride in their ethnic group's concepts when the group is perceived in a negative manner by the wider society. The family has the most impact on the child's identity formation. If the family does not provide the substantive and consistent exposure to racial and cultural frameworks that pertain to the child, his or her self-image will not be minority-oriented.

Zuniga (1991, p. 21) identified another component that interacts with the child's development of awareness of his or her ethnic identity. She defined this ethnic awareness as

the child's understanding of own and other ethnic groups. Awareness involves knowledge about ethnic groups, their critical attributes, characteristics, history, and customs, as well as the difference between oneself and others. It changes with experience, exposure to new information and developing cognitive abilities. . . . Moreover, if the family denies the importance of the child's racial/ethnic identity, consistent communication about that identity will be absent. The child will not have an ethnic awareness or learn how to adapt as a minority child who can value his/her diversity. The child will be unable to utilize a minority cultural system in addition to the majority cultural system or be able to effectively defend against racism.

The NABSW reaffirmed its opposition to transracial placements in a position paper published in 1994. It noted that the issues of transracial adoption are not separate from those of foster care placement. It proposed that the solution to transracial adoption can be found in the development of a systemic approach that utilizes the philosophy of permanency, beginning with efforts to maintain the family before need for placement occurs. Prevention, as a primary tool to avoid foster care placements, would also prevent transracial adoptions. The NABSW also states that "family preservation, reunification and adoption should work in tandem toward finding permanent homes for children" (1994, p. 4). The NABSW argued that too many children are removed from their homes before substantive efforts are made to prevent their removal.

The issue of appropriate placement is critical in that the profile of the adoptive family has changed dramatically from the 1960s. The transracially adoptive families of the 1970s were characterized as well-off financially, highly educated, and politically liberal. They have been supplemented by a group of foster parent adopters who are moderately educated and traditional in terms of family and political values (Rosenthal et al., 1991; Pohl & Harris, 1992). Increasingly, the foster care system is the primary door through which children enter on the way to adoption. In New York State, for example, over 80% of the adoptions are with foster parents.

The NABSW (1994) asserted that institutional racism is inherent in the child welfare system and is manifested in the disproportionate number of minority children removed from their homes as well as the reasons for their removal—the primary reason is for neglect, not abuse. The former is a problem that is exacerbated by the factors of poverty, homelessness, and other societal problems that burden the system. Gray and Nybell (1990, p. 513) support the views of the NABSW. They found that the "literature reflects that African American children come into care more frequently, remain in care longer, and may receive less desirable placements than white children."

Other failures of the system are seen in the lack of adequate resources for family preservation, a workforce that is not reflective of the system's clients, and policies and practices that effectively reinforce barriers. Additional weaknesses are found in the paucity of people of color in management and policymaking positions, and as direct child care workers. Ignorance of cultural differences and lack of cultural sensitivity also contribute obstacles (Gray & Nybell, 1990; Pohl & Harris, 1992; NABSW, 1994). Gray and Nybell (1990) cited studies of the National Child Welfare Training Center, which reported 78% of the workers and 80% of the supervisors are white. The majority had not received in-service training in service provision to African-American families. In addition, high fees for adoption home studies, too inflexible standards, and poor recruitment techniques continue to act as barriers to inrace adoptions for African American and other minority children.

One solution to mitigate these problems, which has been suggested by the NABSW (1994) and instituted by many state departments of social service, is the development of specialized foster care and adoption agencies. These agencies, established and implemented by African-American and other minority groups, provide the culturally relevant programs and culturally knowledgeable staffs to offer services that address the barriers cited in this chapter. As the founding director of such an agency, this author has had direct experience that verifies the success of this approach. The author's agency placed 97% of its black children in African-American homes.

The NABSW (1994, p. 5) cited a North American Council on Adoptable Children study, conducted in 1986, which found that "specialized agencies placed approximately 94% of their 341 black children and 66% of their 38 Hispanic children in same race homes, but the traditional agencies did so only 51% of the time with 806 black children and 30% of the time with their 168 Hispanic children." Additional information from this study indicated that eight traditional agencies placed at least 85% of their children of color transracially.

The creation of specialized programs is a response to the problem that has to interact in concert with other initiatives. Working within the present system, Gray and Nybell (1990) proposed teaching majority staff members using a model of working with African-American families that is based on the premise of a "culturally relevant" rather than "deficit" model. Their model defines concepts of culture, enculturation, and socialization, and incorporates information on African-American culture, history, family, and expressive behaviors. For example, the authors recommend that topics include use of the kinship network, understanding the role that African-American men play as partners (even if they are not physically present in the home) issues of child rearing from a black perspective, language and expressive behavior, understanding black English, and the numerous community resources available as mediating entities and assists to the system.

Finally, an inherent theme at the core of the debate on transracial adoption is the premise that either the pro or con position is "in the child's best interest." Both sides would ultimately argue that their position is more commensurate with the child's best interest. The value and importance of establishing permanency for a child is not the issue here. Both opponents as well as proponents of transracial adoption agree that each and every child needs and deserves a permanent home. *This author would agree with the NABSW and others, who view the placement of children in families of*

the same race and culture as in the child's best interest. The value of ensuring that African-American children learn the whole and complete sum of
who they are, as members of a distinct group, is the issue.

The following statement by the NABSW (1994, p. 5) provides a succinct
summation of the importance of this issue.

Culture is the single most important filter through which we see the world. It is
through culture that we assign the meaning to circumstances, situations, and experiences in our world—it is one's world view. In the African-American community,
culture is the sum total of our historical experience. This includes the impact of
and survival strategies developed from the experience of slavery and racism in
America."

Transracial adoptions continue, as does the debate. Is it time, perhaps,
to broaden the debate on transracial adoption from the issue of what is
"in the child's best interest" to encompass the compelling issue of who
gets to define what *is* "in the child's best interest?"

WORKS CITED

Andujo, E. (1988). Ethnic Identity of transethnically adopted Hispanic adolescents.
    Social Work, 33, 531–535.
Bagley, C. (1993). Transracial adoption in Britain: a follow-up study with policy
    considerations. *Child Welfare, 73* (3), 285–299.
Chestang, L. (1972). The dilemma of biracial adoption. *Social Work* 17 (3), 100–
    115.
Child Welfare League of America. (1968). *Standards for Adoptive Practice.* New
    York: CWLA.
Child Welfare League of America. (1973). *Standards for Adoptive Practice.* New
    York: CWLA.
Child Welfare League of America. (1978). *Standards for Adoptive Practice.* New
    York: CWLA.
Child Welfare League of America. (1988). *Standards for Adoptive Practice.* Wash-
    ington, DC: CWLA.
Child Welfare League of America. (1995). Multiethnic Placement Act of 1994,
    Briefing Paper. Washington, DC: CWLA.
Gray, S. & Nybell, L. (1990). Issues in African-American family preservation.
    Child Welfare, 69 (6), 513–523.
Grow, L. & Shapiro, D. (1974). *Black Children, White Parents: A Study of
    Transracial Adoption.* Washington, DC: CWLA.
Hayes, P. (1993). Transracial adoption: politics and ideology. *Child Welfare* 72 (3),
    301–310.
Helwig, A. & Ruthven, D. (1990). Psychological ramifications of adoption and
    implications for counseling. *Journal of Mental Health Counseling,* 12 (1),
    24–37.
Johnson, P., Shireman, J. & Watson, K. (1987). Transracial adoption and the devel-
    opment of black identity at age eight. *Child Welfare, 66* (1), 45–55.

Jones, C. & Else, J. (1979). Racial and cultural issues in adoption. *Child Welfare*, 58 (6), 373–382.

Kim, D. S. (1977). How they fared in American homes: a follow-up study of adopted Korean children in the United States. *Children Today*, 6, 2–6.

Kim, S., Hong, S. & Kim, B. (1979). Adoption of Korean children by New York area couples: a preliminary study. *Child Welfare*, 58 (7), 419–427.

Ladner, J. A. (1977). *Mixed Families: Adopting Across Racial Boundaries*. New York: Doubleday.

Locke, D. (1992). *Increasing Multicultural Understanding*. Newbury Park, CA: Sage Publications.

McAdoo, H. (Ed.). (1993). *Family Ethnicity*. Newbury Park, CA: Sage Publications.

McRoy, R. & Zurcher, L. (1983). *Transracial and Inracial Adoptees: The Adolescent Years*. Springfield, IL: Charles C. Thomas.

Milner, D. (1983). *Children and Race*. Beverly Hills, CA: Sage Publications.

National Association of Black Social Workers. (1972). Position statement on transracial adoptions. Conference Proceedings, Nashville.

National Association of Black Social Workers. (1994). Position statement: Preserving African-American Families. Detroit: NABSW.

Pohl, C. & Harris, W. (1992). *Transracial Adoption: Children and Parents Speak*. New York: Franklin Watts.

Rosenthal, J., Groze, V., Curiel H. & Westcott, P. (1991). Transracial and inracial adoption of special needs children. *Journal of Multicultural Social Work*, 1 (3), 13–32.

Shireman, J. (1988). *Growing Up Adopted: An Examination of Major Issues*. Chicago: Child Care Society.

Shireman, J. & Johnson, P. (1986). Longitudinal study of black adoption: single parent, transracial and traditional. *Social Work*, 31 (3), 171–176.

Silverman, A. (1993). Outcomes of transracial adoption. *The Future of Children*, 3 (1), 104–118.

Simon R. & Alstein, H. (1977). *Transracial Adoption*. New York: John Wiley.

Simon, R. & Alstein, H. (1981). *Transracial Adoption: A Follow-up*. Lexington, MA: Lexington Books.

Simon, R. & Alstein, H. (1987). *Transracial Adoptees and their Families: A Study of Identity and Commitment*. New York: Praeger.

Spar, K. (1991). Child welfare and foster care reform: Issues for Congress. Washington, DC: Congressional Research Service, Library of Congress.

Zuniga, M. (1991). Transracial adoption: educating the parents. *Journal of Multicultural Social Work*, 1 (2), 7–31.

11

Reproductive Rights: Who Speaks for African-American Women?

Stacey Daniels

The topic of reproductive rights represents an extremely complex set of issues for any woman. For the African-American woman especially, reproductive rights involve issues of feminism, sexuality, procreation, and health in general.

FEMINISM OR WOMANISM?

Since the dawn of the feminist era, black women have been continually asked whether the movement is relevant for us. These probes are usually placed in the context of: Are white women's issues the same as yours? Whether the feminist movement seeks to do so or not, many African-American women have long felt that it does not adequately represent our interests. It does not address sexism within a racist society or other issues specific to black women's circumstances. African-American women are increasingly using the term "womanism" to describe feminism from an Afro-centric perspective. Womanism *is* meant to "express a philosophy that celebrates the black roots and ideals of black life while giving a balanced presentation of black womandom" (Ogunyemi, 1985). The womanist movement emphasizes the unique needs of women of African descent as opposed to the "limitations implicit in the notion of black feminism"

(Hudson-Weems, 1989). Womanism captures the essence of black women's feelings resulting from vestiges of slavery, second-class citizenship through segregation, and subjugation from our own people.

Feminism and womanism both seek to stress the validity of the needs of the individual woman as she defines them. As such, the issue of reproductive rights is viewed broadly, encompassing whatever reproductive choices the woman wants them to encompass.

REPRODUCTION AND CONTRACEPTION

The right to bear children when wanted is a relatively new right for women in terms of available, effective contraceptives. The 35th anniversary of the birth control Pill in 1995 is of more than symbolic importance to women in their assertion of reproductive rights, since the Pill represents a reliable, easy method of controlling fertility. Some 80% of sexually active women have used the Pill at one time or another, because of its ease and effectiveness. Its availability has allowed women to postpone childbearing in efforts to pursue education and professional careers. Public health officials suggest that the ability to reduce and delay childbearing has contributed greatly to women's representation in the workforce today in such a variety of professions (Birth control pill, 1995).

The importance of pregnancy prevention to the future of a woman—her career, better economic conditions for her family, and the realization of personal dreams—cannot be overemphasized. Planning parenthood allows a woman to have children when she is ready for them emotionally and economically, and when she and her family can offer them the best future possible. It allows parenthood not just to be an event that happens, but to become one that is longed for with excitement. It becomes not a potential problem, but a gift or even a blessing. African-American women have these same hopes and dreams for themselves and their families. That African-American women have made the most of controlling their fertility is evidenced by the number of black women who delay childbearing or do not reproduce at all.

It is surprising that contraceptive research has not progressed farther than it has in the mid-1990s. Many pharmaceutical companies have withdrawn from contraceptive research, because it is slow and costly. Developing a new contraceptive may take 25–30 years and cost $50–100 million. When contraceptive research is contemplated, it much more often has women as its focus (Daniels, 1992). The preoccupation with female reproduction and contraception is looked at with some degree of bitterness by some women. Women are an easy, even understandable target for contraceptive researchers; as one said, it is "easier to interfere with one ovum than millions of sperm" (Ford Foundation, 1990). The woman is the visible partner in pregnancy and contraceptive focus on her places responsibility (and blame) for childbearing on her as well. It might occur to women that it may be more productive for them to focus on the power that this gives us, especially the long-sought power over our own bodies.

During the 1990s we have seen greater prevalence of alternative methods of contraception that do not require women to remember to pop a pill every day (and with some of the low-dosage pills, to pop it at roughly the same time each day). Injectables that can last several months (Depo-Provera) and implants that can last several years (Norplant) may have their own side effects, but they are attractive for exactly this reason: they don't require daily attention. Psychologically, this further means that reproduction does not have to occupy some degree of daily attention, elevating it to prominence that may not be appropriate for one's lifestyle. While this freedom is welcomed, on the other hand America continues to exhibit discomfort with suggestions that medical advances such as long-lasting contraceptive implants should be used to prevent adolescent pregnancy.

Of course, availability of contraceptives is also a matter of cost. The Pill, at about $20 for a monthly cycle, may well be beyond the affordability of many women, especially adolescents. The newer contraceptive implants and injectables are even more expensive (implants cost $107 annually over a five-year continuous use period; injectables are $140 per year; Westfall & Main, 1995). Finally, even if the woman has insurance, her plan may not cover birth control methods.

Even though there may be a tendency to assume that "reproductive rights" is mostly about preventing pregnancy, the subject also includes decisions about when to bear children and family size. It's probably safe to say that having a child at some point in their lives is a desire of many, many women, and African-American women are no exception, regardless of income. Conflicting attitudes may exist over the "right" to have children without first having adequate income for their proper sustenance and care before and after birth. Does this mean that a lack of economic resources gives society a "right" to discourage that desire for childbearing? If the decision is a personal one, does society then have the "right" to refuse to contribute to the child's later care? Perhaps paradoxically, Levine and Dubler (1990) suggest that groups that feel threatened seek reproduction as an "affirmation of life and a hope for survival," seeing a "pronatalist" message in religious and secular institutions. Even though black churches are decentralized, largely autonomous, and have seen many of their members move away as they become more economically upscale, they remain a powerful force of influence over the behavior and attitudes of African-Americans. "Doctrinally fundamentalist" and "socially conservative" (Dalton, 1989), African-American churches rarely promote a woman's right to choice. Even if their messages move beyond sexual abstinence outside of marriage and acknowledge the value of contraception, their concern with childbearing has more to do with not having more children than one can personally afford.

As Christopher and Leak (1982) interpret sociobiological thought, "the notion of group advantage in the evolution of individual behavior has been replaced by the concept that natural selection produces organisms whose ultimate concern is genetic self-interest and selfishness." One way that individuals can increase their own genetic success is by accepting a short-term loss for a long-term gain. Vining (1986) observes that a study of modern human populations reveals that, for all but one "unique" period of rising fertility, an inverse relationship actually exists between "reproductive fitness and 'endowment' (i.e., wealth, success, and measured aptitude)." Following these lines of thinking, the sociobiologist might further conclude that those with the greatest potential to contribute to society would also be those most likely to delay childbearing, and are therefore more likely to choose abortion. Does this tendency malserve the future potential of the African-American community? If the decision to delay childbearing eventually becomes a failure to reproduce, is not the future gene pool of African-Americans at risk for dilution? When these considerations are entered into the discussion, it is no wonder that African-Americans emphasize the value of reproduction to us as a people and are less visible advocates of abortion.

Based on analysis of the most recent National Survey of Family Growth, Williams (1994) reports that African-American women were less likely than whites to have a birth that is jointly desired by both partners, they were less likely to know the partner's preference for childbearing, but they were also more likely than white women to have a birth that was wanted by the partner, but not by the woman. Black women reported more births that were wanted by the partner than either wanted by them alone or that was jointly planned. This study strongly suggests that African-American women, perhaps more so than other women, are likely to view childbearing as a way to please a partner and/or solidify a relationship. Zinn (1989) and Wilson (1987) suggest that dynamics may actually exist that encourage childbearing among unmarried African-American women, because of the high rate of unemployed black men.

However, Kost and Forrest (1995) report that African-American women are more likely than Hispanic or white women to say a birth is unwanted, and more often than white women say that a wanted birth was *mistimed*. Such a high degree of unwanted pregnancy may explain why black women account for nearly twice as many abortions as white women.

ABORTION

When the topic "reproductive rights" is raised, abortion must inevitably be discussed. For black women, abortion may be tied up with feelings about genocide, juxtaposed with desires for the same control over one's body afforded women by the *Roe v. Wade* decision of 1973 that legalized abortion in America. The *Roe* decision enhanced the safety of abortion, increased its availability, and reduced its cost because it was no longer a clandestine activity performed by those of questionable qualification. While African-American women share the same goals for maximizing their future potential as all women, fears of a "conspiracy" against African-American procreation complicate blacks' philosophical attitudes toward abortion. Fears about abortion as genocide seem less hysterical when one remembers the forced or coerced sterilization of the past. Nsiah-Jefferson (1989) reports, for example, cases of doctors who would deliver the babies of black Medicaid mothers who agreed to be sterilized. Recent urging of sterilization for AIDS-infected women, who are disproportionately women of color, adds fuel to the genocide perspective (King, 1991).

Abortion may be more of a practical than political decision for African-American women. Black women start families earlier but also stop reproducing earlier than do white women. As they become older, with greater financial resources, they are able to exercise more control over their reproductive lives.

Although African-American women account for nearly twice as many abortions as do white women, we are ambivalent in our support for abortion. An official of the Gallup Organization has been quoted as stating that the "most conservative people on the abortion issue are Blacks, Hispanics, and white Catholics" (Lee & Gold, 1990). Undoubtedly, the church is of great significance in African-American culture. If, as Dalton (1989) asserts, most African-American churches are "socially conservative," it is no wonder that there is a relative lack of visibility of black women advocating for abortion rights. The strong religious environment in which many African-American women were raised may also account for a reticence to discuss sexuality and birth control options openly.

But even if as a group we are inclined to value procreation and believe that sex and abortion are sins, it is clear that our behaviors do not necessarily correspond (Lee & Gold, 1990). Some African-American women use the examples of sterilization as well as slavery's forced childbearing to augment their pro-choice arguments. The important issue for them is choice—the ability to choose for oneself one's reproductive path. During the time of slavery, no woman had good birth control options. Nor did African-American women have the option of saying "no" to the slavemaster's sexual advances. The mulatto progeny that often resulted may have been treated better in terms of duties, but they were also often the target of jealousy and contempt from their darker-hued brothers and sisters. Even today the color-conscious wars rage among black Americans. Is it any wonder that black women would find the ability to choose whether to bear children or not something to be desired?

Abortion sometimes becomes a more attractive option when economic constraints limit the size of family that can be financially supported. But economics more often has the opposite effect of limiting abortion. The rights of poor black women to abortion are limited by cost and state re-strictions, which force them to travel long distances to secure an abortion (Henshaw, 1995). It is especially ironic that the abatement of federal Med-icaid coverage for abortion has been shown actually to be more costly than providing the service. It is readily apparent that the long-term Medic-aid costs associated with prenatal care (when it occurs) and delivery ex-ceed the cost of abortion, without even mentioning the long-term cost to the family and potentially to society of unwanted births. Many poor women who desire an abortion supplant other needs to pay for the proce-dure; for example, in 1993 the average charge for a first-trimester abortion was only about $100 less than the average monthly AFDC benefit. (Alan Guttmacher Institute, 1995) If a woman on welfare wants an abortion, she would have to sacrifice so that many other things (such as utilities and food) may be neglected. Further, since it understandably takes a while to scrape up the nearly $300 cost, by the time the money is secured the woman is likely to be beyond the first trimester, which makes the proce-dure more costly and more dangerous. Some of these restrictions lead to women still choosing illegal abortions. Perhaps surprisingly, illegal abor-tions continue to present a real concern, and today deaths from legal and illegal abortion are more common among women of color (Council Re-port, 1992).

Some also find it dangerously ironic that today's abortion debate is be-ing crafted and led by white males. There are countless psychological ex-planations of these males' anti-choice tendencies. Perhaps their interest is in increasing the supply of "adoptable white babies." Perhaps their goal is punishing the woman who can't say no by condemning her with the child (the child as curse?). It is clear, however, that their goal is control—if no longer control over what a woman does with her body, at least they will exercise a modicum of control over the results of her actions.

SEXUALITY AND ADOLESCENTS

The schizophrenia of black women toward abortion is not difficult to understand—America itself is schizophrenic about sexuality. For example, the fact that the United States has a higher rate of teen pregnancy than other developed nations has been well-documented (Scott-Jones, 1993). It is clear that both black and white adolescent females in America are be-coming sexually active at younger ages. Girls today become sexually ma-ture at relatively young ages (average age of menarche of 12.5, compared to the average of 16.5 in 19th-century Europe; Eveleth, 1986). This bio-logical maturation is not accompanied by psychological maturation, nor by changes in society that accept young people as adults at younger ages. By contrast, they are actually expected to behave as more dependent adolescents, in the homes of their parents, as opposed to beginning to head their own households.

A major difference between African-American and white adolescents who become pregnant can be seen in the greater tendency for white adolescents to be married or get abortions. Cost again contributes to outcome, since black adolescents are less likely to have money for an abortion. Therefore, the black teen's sexuality is more visible and castigated. Even when adolescents of color are omitted from the analysis, the childbearing and abortion rates for America's white teens remains higher than that of other industrialized nations. The increased rates are not due to greater rates of sexual activity, nor does the existence of welfare appear to serve as a greater incentive (some of the comparison countries have more generous welfare policies). Scott-Jones (1993) suggests that a more equitable distribution of income, more health and unemployment benefits, widely available sex education, contraceptives, abortion services, and a more open and accepting attitude toward sexual activity among young people would all contribute to lower rates.

Current social conditions make it generally difficult to become a responsible adult, and developing sexual responsibility is particularly difficult for those making the transition to adulthood. We are plagued with the mysterious and uncontrolled sexually transmitted disease—AIDS. In spite of the life-threatening nature of AIDS, the mass media continue to bombard adolescents with sexual stimuli and sexual themes in all genres, from rock videos to product advertisements (Scott-Jones, 1993, p. 1).

BLACK WOMEN'S HEALTH ISSUES

Black women may also be underrepresented among vocal and visible advocates for abortion because of their concern with wider issues of black women's health (Lee & Gold, 1990). Black women have reduced access to health care, owing to lack of insurance and underinsurance, and challenges to Medicaid will likely result in coverage for fewer families from this source as well. Even for women who are covered by insurance, discrimination exists within the system: women pay more for the same coverage, or cannot buy the same coverage as men (Barber-Madden & Kotch, 1990). Women's difficulty accessing medical insurance affects their children, through restricted access for their children and even before birth through inadequate prenatal care.

Options for accessible, affordable providers (especially in inner cities) continue to be reduced. Cuts in federal scholarships for medical students resulted in a decline of African-American doctors from 26,000 in 1984 to 16,000 in 1990. The reduced availability of black physicians has been accompanied by a decline in the number of African-Americans using private physicians, resulting in minorities using the emergency room as their primary health provider. The emergency room does not perform screenings for breast cancer or Pap smears, nor is the emergency room able to focus on any preventive measures to promote health maintenance. Again, lack of preventive care results in higher long-term costs. In one study in Harlem, over half of the black women who entered the hospital with breast cancer were already incurable, compared to 8% of white women (Gorman, 1991). African-American women have accused feminists and abortion advocates of being myopic in their focus, ignoring these larger issues that must be of concern to Black America.

BLACK WOMEN AND RESEARCH

Actual research and information regarding reproduction and African-American women should command greater attention than the extant literature would suggest has been conducted. Of course, a major reason for the dearth of published research about African-American women and reproduction or sexuality in general involves the abuses that African-Americans have endured at the hands of researchers. These abuses have resulted in suspiciousness toward researchers (usually white) on the part of African-Americans, and an unwillingness to participate in research, especially research that does not include African-Americans among the designers and implementors of the research.

There are valid research needs focusing on African-Americans, and specifically on African-American women. For example, African-Americans and women experience a greater incidence of hypertension and diabetes, disorders that also afflict women in greater numbers than men. Most important are those studies that involve reproductive health and disorders. Black women have a higher incidence of fibrocystic disease, more cervical cancer, and are diagnosed with breast cancer at younger ages than whites. In general, greater knowledge about reproductive disorders of black women and possible ways to prevent them are warranted.

As mentioned earlier, AIDS afflicts more women of color than white women; in 1994 African-American women accounted for 57% of the known AIDS cases among women. The 1994 infection rates were 16 times higher for African-American women than among whites (AIDS in black America, 1995). Since women are at greater risk of getting AIDS from men than vice versa, and it appears that the progression of infection to AIDS is more rapid among women than men (J. L. Mitchell, 1989; Minkoff et al., 1987), it is likewise reasonable to suggest that greater research may indicate if black women have a different susceptibility to the disease and its progression. It has been argued that HIV-infected women, who are the same class of women who have traditionally been encouraged or coerced to limit reproduction on grounds of either benefits to themselves and their families or benefit to society, are now being encouraged to limit reproduction to prevent transmission of disease to their children on grounds of costs to society (Levine & Dubler, 1990). It is again ironic that this perspective is being advocated as "socially and morally responsible" at a time in history when making the choice for termination is becoming more restricted.

CONCLUSION

Finally, what does African-American society say to the African-American woman regarding her reproductive rights and, de facto, her sexuality? African-American culture does not seem to endorse the classic Madonna/ whore dichotomy with the same strength as in the 1950s. Now the crime may not be the sexuality of black women as much as its visibility through pregnancy, especially when unwed and supported by public assistance.

The effects of our sexuality on our young people is inescapable. As the sexual revolution was overtaking America in the 1960s and 1970s, unfortunately, perhaps, adolescents were not isolated from the revolution—they were watching. They continue to watch as we define for ourselves appropriate (adult) sexual behavior and relationships. Whether unfair or not, the black woman's definition of sexual norms is more visible to our young people, because they most often live with and are reared by us. In our quest for psychosexual health, have we made such a case for the naturalness of sex as we define it that our standards (or perhaps relaxed standards) have become the norm for our young people?

We are aware that adolescence is a time during which the developmental task is to decide one's identity, and begin to approach the future adult persona through experimentation with what are perceived as expected adult behaviors. Are we caught in a dilemma produced by adolescents mimicking what they *perceive* we think is appropriate adult behavior?

But beyond the sexuality of young people, does African-American society accept the sexuality and reproductive rights of African-American women? "Nice" black women can enjoy their sexuality; aren't we supposed to do so to be complete, real women? If so, heterosexual African-American men and women are likely to have multiple and "riskier" partners (especially among the unmarried). Peterson et al. (1993) suggest that the fewer black males than females in the pool of eligible marriage partners means that married black males may be less likely than married black females to be monogamous. Therefore, they further state, barrier methods of contraception are essential for black women if strategies are not discovered which convince black men to not choose multiple partners. Women are expected to be the one in charge of sexual responsibility. But as social psychologist Albert Bandura (1987) observes (cited in Dalton, 1989), where pregnancy prevention alone allows women to exercise independent control, use of condoms requires women to exercise control over the behavior of men. So we are even given tips on how to communicate effectively with our partners to convince them to wear condoms. And one of the few new advances in reproductive technology in the 1990s is the *female condom* which, at a cost of about $3 each is even less effective than the male condom and is probably the least effective contraceptive device option available (AIDS in black America, 1995; Mitchell, 1995).

So are these reproductive rights? The low-dosage Pill, contraceptive implants and injectables, and the female condom all represent advances in allowing reproductive self-determination. But it would be nice to see increased advances in male contraceptive technology, even if we can't control their use to our benefit.

And do we even need our own voice, a separate voice? Perhaps abortion as an issue has not resonated as clearly in the black community because we need a voice less for reproductive limitation. We seek voices for our true reproductive choice—voices affirming our right to *responsibly* bear children or not bear children. I think it is imperative that this voice must always insert the word *responsible* in the conversation, for it neither advances us as individuals nor as a people to reproduce without consideration for ensuring that our fruit has the best chance to become filled with pride and to receive opportunities for greater success than that of any generation before them. So who speaks for the African-American woman? I say it's our progeny—and the fact that they speak to us is more important than who speaks for us.

WORKS CITED

AIDS in black America: it's not just a gay thing. (1995). *Crisis,* 102 (5), 34–35.

Alan Guttmacher Institute. (1995). The cost implications of including abortion coverage under Medicaid. *Issues in Brief,* March.

Barber-Madden, R. & Kotch, J. B. (1990). Maternity care financing: Universal access or universal care? *Journal of Health Politics, Policy, and Law,* 15 (4), 797–813.

Birth control pill turns 35 years old. (1995). *Jet,* 88 (2), 16.

Christopher, S. B. & Leak, G. (1982). Evolutional logic and Adlerian social interest. *Psychological Reports,* 52 (2), 375–378.

Council Report. (1992). Induced termination of pregnancy before and after Roe v. Wade: Trends in the mortality and morbidity of women. *Journal of the American Medical Association,* 268 (22), 3231–3239.

Dalton, H. L. (1989). AIDS in blackface. *Daedalus,* 188 (3), 205–227.

Daniels, S. (1992). Women's health issues. In L. H. Talbott, E. Noble & L. G. Klein eds., *Women in the Heart of America: Concerns, Needs and Priority Issues for the 1990s.* The Women's Foundation of Greater Kansas City, MO.

Eveleth, P. B. (1986). Timing of menarche: Secular trends to population differences.

In J. B. Lancaster & B. A. Hamburg eds., *School-age Pregnancy and Parenthood*. New York: Aldine, 39–52.

Ford Foundation. (1990). *Reproductive Health: A Strategy for the 90s*. New York: Ford Foundation.

Henshaw, S. K. (1995). Factors hindering access to abortion services. *Family Planning Perspectives*, 27 (2), 54–59.

Hudson-Weems, C. (1989). Cultural and agenda conflicts in academia: Critical issues for African women's studies. *Western Journal of Black Studies*, 13 (4), 185–189.

King, P. A. (1991). Helping women helping children: Drug policy and future generations. *Milbank Quarterly*, 69 (4), 595–627.

Gorman, C. (1991). Why do blacks die young? *Time*, 138 (11), 50–52.

Kost, K. & Forrest, J. D. (1995). Intention status of U.S. births in 1988: Differences by mothers' socioeconomic and demographic characteristics. *Family Planning Perspectives*, 27 (1), 11–17.

Lee, F. R. & Gold, R. B. (1990). Empty womb: Black women's views on abortion. *Essence*, 21 (1), 51–52.

Levine, C. D. & Dubler, N. (1990). Uncertain risks and bitter realities: The reproductive choices of HIV-infected women. *Milbank Quarterly*, 68 (3), 321.

Minkoff, H. et al. (1987). Pregnancies resulting in infants with acquired immunodeficiency syndrome or AIDS related complex: Follow-up of mothers, children and subsequent born siblings. *Obstetrics and Gynecology*, 69, 288–291.

Mitchell, J. L. (1989). Drug abuse and AIDS in women and their affected offspring. *Journal of the American Medical Association*, 81, 841–842.

Mitchell, M. (1995). Personal Communication, May.

Nsiah-Jefferson, L. (1993). Access to reproductive genetic services for low income women and women of color. *Fetal Diagnosis Therapy*, 8, Supplement 1, 1-2–127.

Ogunyemi, C. O. (1985). Womanism: The dynamics of the contemporary black female novel in English. *Signs: Journal of Women in Culture and Society*, 11 (1), 63–80.

Peterson, J. L., Catania, J. A., Dolcini, M. M. & Faigeles, B. (1993). Multiple sexual partners among blacks in high-risk cities. *Family Planning Perspectives*, 25 (6), 257–262.

Scott-Jones. D. (1993). Adolescent childbearing: Whose problem? What can we do? *Phi Delta Kappan*, 75 (3), 1–12.

Vining, D. R. (1986). Social versus reproductive success: The central theoretical problem of human sociobiology. *Behavioral and Brain Sciences* 9 (1), 167–216.

Westfall, J. M. & Main, D. S. (1995). The contraceptive implant and the injectable: A comparison of costs. *Family Planning Perspectives*, 27 (1), 34–36.

Williams, L. B. (1994). Determinants of couple agreement in U.S. fertility decisions. *Family Planning Perspectives*, 26 (4), 169–173.

Wilson, W. J. (1987). *The Truly Disadvantaged: The Inner City, the Underclass and Public Society*. Chicago: University of Chicago Press.

Zinn, M. B. (1989). Family, race and poverty in the eighties. *Signs: Journal of Women in Culture and Society*, 14, 856–874.

12

The Roots of Coping Behavior for African-American Women: A Literary Perspective

Imani Lillie B. Fryar

There are cultural variations in how individuals of different societies handle oppression. Strategies appearing negative to the outside observer may be the appropriate mechanism for the oppressed to repossess or reconnect to their cultural bearings. When African-American women were enslaved, various stereotypes were created to define and control their behavior, such as mammy, sapphire, Caldonia, sex-kitten, and so on. However, through literary analysis, I will examine works of African-American women from various time periods to illuminate the strategies these women elected as survival techniques, redefining themselves along the way, and how these coping skills are residuals of the African tradition. Some of the works cited are: *Our Nig,* Harriet Wilson; *Incidents in the Life of a Slave Girl,* Linda Brent; *Their Eyes Were Watching God,* Zora Neal Hurston; *Sula,* Toni Morrison; and *Waiting to Exhale,* Terry McMillan. Lena Wright Myers in her research, *Black Women Do They Cope Better* (1991, p. 14) states:

Theoretically, it is believed that we learn to think of ourselves as we do, primarily on the basis of how others see us, as shown by their behavior toward us. But not all others count equally. Those people who have the most impact upon our self-esteem and attitudes are those we have the most in common with. Our key to coping with racism and sexism . . . was to get an image of ourselves based on how well we do whatever we are doing, and how others whose opinions matter to us view our success in whatever we do.

RELIGION AND RITUALS FOR COPING

For black women it would be, of course, other black women/mother substitutes. In Myers' report, she interviewed 200 black women from Grand Rapids, Michigan, in 1972; 200 from Jackson, Mississippi, in 1974; and 200 women ten years later from Georgia, Washington, D.C., Illinois, Michigan, Mississippi, and New Jersey. The women interviewed attested to a strong religious connection:

Not only have family ties been a source of strength for black women, but also the church and the clergy. Since slavery, the church has been a viable institution in the lives of black people. The views of the black women in my sample support this contention. The majority of the women felt that the church and religion helped to prepare them for getting ahead in life.

Responses as to how the church and religion helped them included: "The Lord would always show me the way to go." "Got to have something to believe in, in order to get ahead, and I believe in spiritual things" (Myers, 1991, p. 28).

While Myers' work alludes to W.E.B. Du Bois' (1969) theory of living within the veil, "always seeing ourselves through the eyes of others," black women in their coping mechanisms have extracted the "others" to be those whom they trust and who know them. So the veil is a positive covering of protection and is important because, as seekers of the truth, they know that those with whom they have spent time and are like them know them the best. In the African tradition, the highest motivation for individuals is to know their life purpose and pursue it. People in your community know your purpose also.

In the audio book *We Have No Word for Sex,* by Malidoma and Sonofu Some (1994), they talk about the ritual that women have of returning once a year with their rites-of-passage initiates to rebond and nurture one another. Sonofu is from the Dagara tribe of Burkina Faso, West Africa. Her name means "keeper of the rituals" and she describes the many gender-specific rituals. Even in the villages, women and men do not sleep together. Women are constantly bonding and learning how to be women from their elders and female relatives; their abilities are reinforced and nurtured by other women. So when they return to the village to carry out those roles, they are fortified and strong.

In the South it was relatively easy to carry out these traditions in agricultural settings, but with industrialization and continued racist and sexist oppression, it became increasingly difficult for black women to replicate these rituals, and therefore they become isolated. The bond was broken during slavery and black women have not completely found their way back yet. However, the many black female groups such as AKAs, Links, 100 Black Women, Jack & Jill, and International Black Women's Congress, to name a few, all serve to help alleviate the pain of isolation, and they are successful. Nevertheless, it is still important to see the connection these groups have to African traditions so that cultural ties will be strong.

In Linda Brent's *Incident in the Life of a Slave Girl* (1973), Linda's grandmother protected her, most of the time, from the slave master's sexual exploitation. As she ponders her daily battles with Dr. Flint she reflects:

I longed for someone to confide in. I would have given the world to have laid my head on my grandmother's faithful bosom, and told her all my troubles. But Dr. Flint swore he would kill me if I was not silent as the grave. Then, although my grandmother was all in all to me, I feared her as well as loved her . . . she was usually very quiet in her demeanor, but if her indignation was once roused, it was not easily quelled. . . . But even though I did not confide in my grandmother and even evaded her vigilant watchfulness and inquiry, her presence in the neighborhood was some protection to me (p. 28).

Linda had another protector, her great-aunt: "At night I slept by the side of my great-aunt, where I felt safe. He was too prudent to come into her room. She was an old woman and had been in the family for many years" (p. 3).

The paradoxes of the slave system were many. Young girls were exploited, older female slaves were sometimes protected, mostly for their role of experienced caretakers. There was a myriad of ways mothers, grandmothers, aunts, and friends protected the female slave when possible: negotiating to buy their freedom, infanticide, succumbing to sexual exploitation, and death or murder, if necessary, to offer some relief. The will to survive was ever-present.

In addition, in resisting the will of the slave master and other oppressive tactics of the system, the black females would often turn to the residues of their African culture. Africans are a very spiritual people; they have always believed in a higher being than themselves. Their strong belief in spiritual strength is manifested many ways in times of stress. Linda Brent tells about her assurance after praying for her children, husband, family, home, and friends. Although being forbidden to assemble, the strength that her deep abiding faith engendered demonstrates, broadly, an African tradition.

In Kesha Yvonne Scott's *The Habit of Surviving* (1991), she calls upon black women to develop new strategies, because the future generations are asking different questions. Too long have we been surviving in isolation. The healing rituals so prevalent in African communities are absent in American society, and we have been striving to operate without them; reinventing ourselves again and again:

The beginning of the task is to reconsider the way we think about gender based analysis of the social, cultural, racial, sexual, and heterosexist exploitation of black women as blacks, women, and Americans. The beginning of the task is to acknowledge the limitations of conventional thought in these areas. The beginning of the task is to create the safety for black women to cry, to make the movement inside, to jar the survival instincts and spiritual intuition. Then we can model for other women a truly revolutionary process and frame our own social action around our own agenda for personal and political change (p. 228).

This is hard work and we have paid, and are still paying, the price with increased heart attacks, depression, addictions, and various other maladies. We can no longer just save ourselves or our communities; our African roots show us how to do both, and we must repossess these skills. In *Sisters of the Yam,* bell hooks (1993, p. 161) talks about the need for communities of resistance being the healing place for black people. We see such a community created by Sula and Nel, by their friendship, in Toni Morrison's *Sula* (1973).

Except for an occasional leadership role with Sula, Nel had no aggression. Her parents had succeeded in rubbing down to a dull glow any sparkle or sputter within her. Only with Sula did that quality have free rein, but their friendship was so close they, themselves, had difficulty distinguishing one's thoughts from the other's. They never quarreled, those two, the way some girlfriends did over boys, or competed against each other for them. In those days a compliment to one was a compliment to the other; and cruelty to one was a challenge to the other (p. 72).

This passage points out the need for intimacy and its liberating results. Nel could live out her fantasies through Sula, who always did what she wanted to do, regardless of restrictions; she felt nurtured and safe. This safety is similar to instances where African women bonded together in ways that were empowering. There is so much that is misunderstood about African spirituality, but the connection with ancestry is always one of guidance and deeper understanding. The inhuman treatment of slaves at this time caused many to turn to the familiar for guidance, a way of repossessing cultural values. Steve Biko in his essay, "Some African Cultural Concepts" (1993, p. 87), states: "We had our community of saints. We believed—and this was consistent with our views of life—that all people who died had a special place next to God. We felt that a communication with God could only be through these people."

Linda Brent uses this resource in her times of peril:

For more than ten years I had frequented this spot, but never had it seemed to me so sacred as now. A black stump, at the head of my mother's grave, was all that remained of a tree my father had planted. His grave was marked by a small wooden board, bearing his name, the letters of which were nearly obliterated. I knelt down and kissed them, and poured forth a prayer to God for guidance and support in a perilous step I was about to take. As I passed the wreck of the old meeting house where, before Nat Turner's time, the slaves had been allowed to meet for worship, I seemed to hear my father's voice come from it, bidding me not to tarry till I reached freedom or the grave, I rushed on with renovated hopes. My trust in God had been strengthened by that prayer among the graves (p. 93).

Black women would never have been able to survive under the perils of the slave system in America had it not been for their creativity in survival and coping skills. Through literature, we can see a myriad of examples. Relying upon oral tradition, black women have relished in female griots (tribal musician-entertainers) and sister talks they have not always bothered to write down. However, the connections were ways of confirming tactics of resisting alien values and cultures. Picture the babies who were thrown off the slave ships because the mothers did not want to subject their children to the dehumanization of that kind of life. Even after being born in the system, mothers sought ways to protect their children and themselves. In Toni Morrison's *Beloved* (1987), the mother is tormented by the ghost of the child she chose to destroy, not because she was not loved, but because she was beloved. There are a host of other examples, but the main reason these women resisted is that they understood that there had to be a better way. Handling pain can sap one's creative strength, causing confusion and reliance upon unorthodox methods. In Africa, girls are encouraged to endure the pain of the clitoridectomy because it is symbolic of withstanding all the trials and tribulations of life. John S. Mbiti states, in *African Religions and Philosophy* (1969, p. 120):

The physical pain, which the children are encouraged to endure, is the beginning of training them for difficulties and suffering that will come later in life. Endurance of physical and emotional pain is a great virtue among Akamba people, as indeed it is among other Africans, since life in Africa is surrounded by much pain from one source or another.

CONTEMPORARY COPING METHODS

Terry McMillan's contemporary novel *Waiting To Exhale* (1992) offers insight into the plight and stress of urban America. Four women, all different in their perceptions of life, but able to cling to one another because of solid acceptance. They took care of one another whenever there was a need. After having a heart attack,

Gloria heard other familiar voices—Bernadine, Savannah, and Robin. Now it seemed like everybody was rubbing different parts of her body; her legs, feet, arms and shoulders. But her feet were still cold. Why were her feet so cold? . . ."I think we're all responsible for her," Bernadine said. "She's our sister. Please tell us

she's going to be all right." The doctor looked at all three women. He knew Bernadine was lying. But, he was use to this (p. 396).

A study by Mary Beth Snapp (1992) of 100 black women and 100 white
women in the Memphis, Tennessee, area on occupational stress, showed
that middle-class black women received more social support than those of
working-class, white women. This story depicts this reality in that black
women seem to seek out the necessary stress relievers to fit their particular
situation.

These questions were asked of the women in the study: "Do levels of
occupational stress and social support for one's career from family, friends
and co-workers vary by race, class background, supervisory status, marital
status and parental status?" "What are the relationships among social
structure, occupational stress, social support and depression?" The findings indicate that

the black women from middle class backgrounds report much higher levels of family support, on the average, than the other groups of women. One may speculate
that because many of the parents of these black women were upwardly mobile,
they may be better providers of social support, appreciating the hard work required to overcome racial obstacles on the job, understanding their daughters' professional or managerial careers, and wanting to give their children the support they
may have lacked for their own careers (p. 51).

In McMillan's *Waiting to Exhale* we see the mothers in the story being
very supportive and concerned with the lives of their daughters, who were
all professionals. Black motherhood has served to increase the strength of
black women; their mothers know the way and are not modest in passing
this information on to their daughters. Sometimes it is the arrangement of
protection, as in the case of Janie Crawford in Zora Neal Hurston's *Their
Eyes Were Watching God,* or it may be the stern instruction Maya Angelou remembers receiving in *I Know Why the Caged Bird Sings,* when her
mother insisted that she nurture her child even though she was a child
herself. Black mothers had to teach their daughters about life because they
were their primary teachers. Angelou talks about the will to survive:

The black female is assaulted in her tender years by all those common forces of
nature at the same time that she is caught in the tri-partite crossfire of masculine
prejudice, white illogical hate and black lack of power. The fact that the adult
American Negro female emerges a formidable character is often met with amaze-
ment, distaste and even belligerence. It is seldom accepted as an inevitable outcome
of struggle won by survivors and deserves respect if not enthusiastic acceptance (p.
231).

In critiquing this work, Joanne M. Braxton, in *Black Women Writing
Autobiography* (1989), believes that Angelou's coping mechanism was a

direct result of the community of black women who nurtured her, building her self-confidence through cultural traditions (p. 197). Because of this, Braxton believes that a triple consciousness exists for the black woman because "she knows who she is, where she comes from and what the source of her strength has been" (p. 13). This knowledge comes most commonly from gender-specific instances, like the friendships described by Terry McMillan. Bernadette, one of the protagonists of *Waiting To Exhale,* began to recount parts of her life after her husband told her that he wanted a divorce to marry a white woman. She realized that she had given up her personal power for him and their children, and when she began to resist, their relationship deteriorated. Her hairdresser suggested that she get involved in something worthwhile:

She belonged to Black Women on the Move, a support group that held workshops for women who wanted to do more with their lives than cook, clean and take care of the kids; for women who weren't moving, but wanted to move; for women who had already achieved some measure of success, but wanted to find a better way to deal with the stress that came with it; for women who wanted to be more than role models, who were willing to make the time to do something for black folks whose lives, for whatever reason, were in bad shape (p. 32).

Communalism is part of the African tradition and was effective, and remains so, as explained in Paula Gidding's book, *When and Where I Enter* (1984, p. 7). She explains the difference between white and African-American female groups:

Black women, many of them cramped for lack of opportunity, had frustrations too. But theirs were based on problems of the race rather than those of their particular class. The black women activists did not have to be altruistic to have this perspective. The fact was, they understood that their fate was bound with that of the masses.

Being bound with the masses also meant that the masses would not always understand one's longings. Therefore, African-American women cope, sometimes, by silence and waiting. Hurston paints Janie Crawford as one who waited for self-fulfillment and love, but her spirituality helped her to persevere:

Her image of Jody tumbled down and shattered. But looking at it she saw that it never was the flesh and blood figure of her dreams. Just something she had grabbed up to drape her dreams over. In a way she turned her back upon the image where it lay and looked further. She had no more blossomy openings dusting pollen over her man, neither any glistening fruit where the petals used to be. She found that she had a host of thoughts she had never expressed to him, and numerous emotions she had never let Jody know about. Things packed up and put away in parts of her heart where she could never find them. She was saving up feelings for some man she had never seen. She had an inside and an outside now, and suddenly she knew how not to mix them (p. 68).

However, in her waiting there is sporadic comforting from Phoebe, a friend who serves as the audience for the story, and by another woman who expresses empathy with her situation:

Janie went down and the landlady made her drink some coffee with her because she said her husband was dead, and it was bad to be having your morning coffee by yourself. "Yo' husband gone tuh work dis mornin', Mis' Woods? Ah seen him go out uh good while uh go. Me and you kin be comp'ny for one 'nother, can't us?" "Oh yes, indeed, Mis' Samuels. You puts me in de mind uh mah friend back in Eatonville. Yeah, you'se nice and friendly jus' lak her" (p. 112).

Friendship has always been a very important part of the lives of females, but for black women especially so, and in this instance we see the selectivity of Janie Crawford, which illustrates that all friends are not equal. Friendships are also forged by black women in order to write, as Hurston aligned herself with philanthropist Mrs. Rufus Osgood Mason to underwrite her research, and Harriet Wilson used Maria Childs to confirm her abilities as a writer in her book.

WRITING AND COPING

Writing is also another way of coping for women/black women, and providing a way of economic support for children. While, early on, the art of writing was the primary quest of males, women had to find a way to uncover their voices. During the abolitionist period, black women had to endure racism and sexism as it pertains to writing. In the slave narratives, their voices had to be authenticated by white women and men, but they continued to speak through autobiographies, travel journals, poems, newspaper articles, and speeches. One of the main concerns of these women was the welfare of their children. Harriet Wilson, on the first page of her introduction to *Our Nig* (1983, p. xii), writes:

In offering to the public the following pages, the writer confesses her inability to minister to the refined and cultivated the pleasure supplied by abler pens. It is not for such these crude narrations appear. Deserted by kindred, disabled by failing health, I am forced to some experiment which shall aid me in maintaining myself and child without extinguishing this feeble life.

The sorrow song aesthetic comes forth in this appeal to the higher level of the public consciousness. While the tone is distressed, it is not hopeless. Writing was a way of coping and, at the same time, continuing to move forward for Wilson. The sorrow song tone of writing demonstrates the way the slave narratives used Christianity to balance insult and truth. One needed the support of the white audience, while at the same time it was necessary for society to hear the clear voice of slavery. In this regard also, writing was cathartic.

Looking at women in Africa, it is evident that they were not always lauded for their accomplishments, even though they may have been lofty. However, they were never deterred from moving toward goals of freeing other women. In Patricia W. Romero's *Life Histories of African Women* (1991), she outlines the lives of seven women from various geographical regions, classes, and lifestyles, suffering the peculiar cultural limits of their era, yet maintaining the dignity and perseverance needed to raise children, establish schools for girls, and break cultural barriers when deemed necessary. In Beverly Mack's chapter, "Hajiya Ma'daki: A Royal Hausa Woman," we see the transitional changes in the Nigerian government and its effect on women. Ma'daki is the granddaughter of a non-Muslim Ha'be slave, daughter of a royal concubine, and became royal wife to a devout Fulani emir (known for political and religious authority). She became acquainted also with central figures in the British colony who were shapers of the lives of her people, such as Captain Frederick Lugard and Flora Shaw. Even though the ancient customs of political and cultural power readily relegated to women were abandoned with the Muslim Fulani influence, Hajiya Ma'daki used her cloak in resisting the status quo and established a school for girls. Education has always been the key for liberation in the eyes of Africans and African-Americans.

Ma'daki's life spanned the period from strict Hausa customs to Muslim practices, and then accommodated Western technology, yet she was able to cope consistently:

Hajiya Ma'daki's life has spanned these significant historical, political and social spheres of influence since her birth, which almost coincided with the arrival of the British in Northern Nigeria. A daughter of Kano royalty, she soon became a royal wife in the nearby emirate of Katsina, thus in her life time officially representing each of two historically rival emirates. During her formative years as a young wife in Katsina, Hajiya Ma'daki witnessed her husband Dikko's concerted efforts to cooperate with the British colonists as they sought to control Northern Nigeria through indirect rule. Although colonial records are silent on the matter, Ma'daki is known to have been a trusted confidante of both Nigerian and British officials who welcomed her advice on various topics. It is clear that her husband, the Emir of Katsina, Alhaji Muhammadu Dikko, valued her perspective on events as well as her company, taking her with him during his travels (p. 53).

One of the great confusions of the slave system for black women had to be the cruel role they were cast into, coming from a system of respect and concern to one of inhumanity. Although Africans are transitioning in many ways to Western ideals, the positive role of African motherhood prevails.

Roots were so important that coming out of the slavery system to free-dom often cast black women in a momentary state of confusion. They were sustained by the female literary artists. Yet it is the period of the Harlem Renaissance and its strong mulatta influence that seemed to cause so much suffering and feelings of abandonment for female artists. It is not just the fact of one's color that is the primary irritant, but how one per-ceives that color. One might surmise that when one is disconnected from cultural roots, albeit briefly, one becomes confused and disoriented. For African and African-American women, it has always been the sense of community, in its many forms, that has sustained them.

Nella Larsen's two novels, *Quicksand* (1928) and *Passing* (1929), show the futile lives of marginal women, who are products of the slave past, trapped in skin that is supposed to represent privilege, but not sufficiently pure. Helga Crane is the heroine in *Quicksand,* a middle-class professional who does not fit in, not in the southern town where she is a schoolteacher, not in Europe with some of her relatives, where she is looked upon as exotic, and not safely in her own skin, which is a constant reminder of her discontentedness. She ends up marrying a black preacher and settling for a life of emptiness. Helga Crane opted not for growth and struggle, but defeat. She assumes this too easily. She visits her white uncle after leaving her teaching position in the South and finds a not-too-friendly reception from his wife:

"Mr. Nilssen has been very kind to you, supported you, sent you to school. But you mustn't expect anything else. And you mustn't come here anymore. It, well, frankly, it isn't convenient. I'm sure an intelligent girl like yourself can understand that." . . . [However, her intelligence did not alleviate her sense of rejection.] Her only impulse was to get as far away from her uncle's house and this woman, his wife, who so plainly wished to disassociate herself from the outrage of her very existence. She was torn with mad fright, an emotion against which she knew but two weapons—to kick and scream or flee (p. 202).

Quicksand can be a metaphor for no foundation and spiritual death. When black women are estranged from their foundation/roots, they are unable to cope. Helga Crane is a woman who is rejected by her white mother and family, and never resolves this pain of abandonment. As a result, she is unable to fit in any environment. She ends up marrying a black preacher, having babies, and resigning herself to a lifetime of unhap-piness. She has no coping skills. Jessie Redmond Fauset, one of the other black female writers of that Harlem Renaissance period, wrote four nov-els—*There Is Confusion* (1924), *Plum Bun* (1929), *The Chinaberry Tree* (1931), and *Comedy American Style* (1931), plus many short stories, arti-cles, and poems. Her theme of "passing" took on another dimension; she was more interested in using upper-middle-class blacks to prove to whites that, with hard work and perseverance, blacks could also make great strides. However, the heroines are narrow and frustrated. Laurentine Strange, the heroine in *The Chinaberry Tree* is the product of an ex-slave, Aunt Saul, and her former master, Captain Halloway; they love each other passionately. At the same time that she is admired as the most beautiful woman in the town, she is also alienated because of her parents' strange and unusual coupling. She can never be totally accepted. In her introduction, Fauset, who is middle class, knows how the system treats blacks and how they feel about their heritage. She imagines the strivings of the black male:

Finally he started out as a slave but he rarely thinks of that. To himself he is a citizen of the United States whose ancestors came over not along with the emigrants of the Mayflower, it is true, but merely a little earlier in the good year, 1619. His forbearers are to him quite simply the early settlers who played a pretty large part in making the land grow. He boasts no Association of the Sons and Daughters of the Revolution, but knows that as a matter of fact and quite inevitably his sons and daughters date their ancestry as far back as any. So quite naturally as his white compatriots he speaks of his "old Boston families," "old Philadelphians," "old Charlestonians." And he has a wholesome respect for family and education and labor and the fruits of labor. He is still sufficiently conservative to lay a slightly greater stress on the first two of these four. Briefly, he is a dark American who wears his joy and rue very much as does the white American. He may wear it with some differences, but it is the same joy and the same rue. So in spite of other intentions I seem to have pointed a moral (p. x).

So the tragic mulatta and her estrangement from her roots represents the embryonic state of the black woman's quest for another kind of literacy. How can she articulate this extreme experience? Earlier, Robert Stepto (1979), in his article "Narration, Authentication, and Authorial Control in Frederick Douglas' Narratives of 1845," defined the quest for literacy and freedom as the primary focus of the 19th-century African-American novels. The early 20th century could represent the quest for identity, as black women became more fully aware of their sexual, as well as racial, limitations. Because Janie Crawford, in Hurston's *Their Eyes Were Watching God,* did not become involved in the trappings of the mulatta syndrome, she was able to return to her roots, fully assured of her strength, telling her story to her friend Phoebe.

It is in later writings that we see this identity evolve more fully with Gwendolyn Brooks winning the Pulitzer Prize for *Annie Allen* in 1950, and others developing themes away from the issues surrounding the mulatta. Maya Angelou, Niki Giovanni, Toni Morrison, Alice Walker, and others are some of the forces who helped usher in another renaissance around the time of the Civil Rights Movement, and beyond.

The writings around the period and beyond have black women defining themselves in creative ways. Alice Walker's (1983) coinage of a black feminist as "womanist" is revealing:

Womanist—1. From womanish (opp. of "girlish", i.e., frivolous, irresponsible, not serious). A black feminist or a feminist of color. From the black folk expression of mothers to female children, "you acting womanish," i.e., like a woman. Usually referring to outrageous audacious, courageous or *willful* behavior. Wanting to know more and in greater depth than is considered "good" for one. Interested in grown-up doings. Acting grown-up. . . Responsible. In charge. *Serious.* . . 3. Loves music. Loves dance. *Loves* the moon. *Loves* the spirit. Loves love and food and roundness. Loves struggle. *Loves* the folk. Loves herself, regardless. 4. Womanist is to feminist as purple to lavender. (xi, xii)

Womanist also serves to describe "sass" as a survival tactic of the black female.

"Mama, I'm walking to Canada and I'm taking you and a bunch of other slaves with me." Reply, "It wouldn't be the first time" (xi).

Sass can be seen in a number of women's writings—Toni Morrison's *Sula* and Walker's Sophie in *The Color Purple*. However, the classic example is Janie Crawford in Hurston's *Their Eyes Were Watching God,* who always maintained a sense of herself through three husbands. The turning point in the novel was the day her husband tried to humiliate her in front of others in the store and her response:

What's de matter wid you no how? You ain't no young girl to be gettin' all insulted' bout yo' looks.

Naw Ah ain't no young gal no mo' but den Ah ain't no old woman neither. Ah reckon Ah looks mah age too. But Ah'm uh woman every inch of me, and Ah know it. Dat's uh whole lot more'n you kin say. You big bellies round here and put out a lot of brag, but 'tain't nothin' to it but yo' big voice. Humph! Talkin' 'bout me lookin' old! When you pull down yo' britches you look lak de change uh life (p. 75).

Sass was definitely a way of coping with the pains of life for black women. The literary criticism about and by black female writers is revealing, as they have learned how to cope better, and have passed it on, in the African tradition. They have coped by relishing in what they feel they do best, not what others have said. The 600 black women in the Myers (1991) study confirmed this in their responses and the conclusions:

When I speak of self-esteem and coping, again I mean self-esteem → coping. I am talking about a feeling of self-worth—a feeling that we are *good enough*. Good enough to and for whom? We are good enough to and for ourselves, our families (who count so much in our lives), and our social support systems, whose experiences are similar and whose opinions matter to us more than any others. We simply feel that we are persons of worth and respect ourselves for what we are. We do not need to be told what we should do or with whom we should identify in order to feel *good enough* about ourselves (p. 61).

Life imitates art and black women have plenty of art to rely upon. They cope by repossessing their roots in a myriad of ways and occasions, not because others say so, but because they know that it is the only way to return to wholeness.

WORKS CITED

Angelou, M. (1969). *I Know Why the Caged Bird Sings*. New York: Random House.

Biko, Steven. (1993). Some African Cultural Concepts. In Teresa M. Redd, ed., *Revelations*. Needham Heights, MA: Ginn.

Braxton, J. M. (1989). *Black Women Writing Autobiography*. Philadelphia: Temple University Press.

Brent, L. (1973). *Incidents in the Life of a Slave Girl*. New York: Harcourt Brace Jovanovich.

Du Bois, W.E.B. (1969). *The Souls of Black Folk*. New York: New-American Library.

Fauset, J.R. (1931). "Foreword" to *The Chinaberry Tree*. New York: Frederick A. Stokes, p. x.

Giddings, P. (1984). *When and Where I Enter*. New York: Bantam Books.

hooks, b. (1993). *Sisters of the Yam*. Boston: South End Press.

Hurston, Z. (1990). *Their Eyes Were Watching God*. New York: Harper & Row.

Larsen, N. (1928). *Quicksand*. New York: Alfred A. Knopf.

Larsen, N. (1929). *Passing*. New York: Alfred A. Knopf.

Mbiti, J. (1969). *African Religions and Philosophy*. Portsmouth, NH: Heinemann.

McMillan, Terry. (1992). *Waiting to Exhale*. New York: Viking Press.

Morrison, Toni. (1973). *Sula*. New York: Alfred A. Knopf.

Morrison, Toni. (1987). *Beloved*. New York: Alfred A. Knopf.

Myers, L. W. (1991). *Black Women Do they Cope Better?* San Francisco: Mellen Research University Press.

Romero, P. (ed.). (1991). *Life Histories of African Women*. London: The Ashfield Press.

Scott, K. Y. (1991). *The Habit of Surviving*. New York: Ballantine Books.

Snapp, M. (1992). Occupational stress, social support, and depression among black and white professional-managerial women. *Women and Health,* 18 (1).

Some, Malidoma and Sobonfu. (1994). *We Have No Word For Sex*. California: Oral Traditions Archives.

Stepto, Robert B. (1979). Narration, authentication, and authorial control in Frederick Douglas' Narratives of 1895. In Dexta Fisher and Robert Stepto, eds.,

Afro-American Literature. New York: Modern Language Association of America.

Walker, A. (1983). *In Search of Our Mother's Gardens.* San Diego: Harcourt Brace Jovanovich.

Wilson, H. (1983). *Our Nig.* New York: Random House.

Epilogue

African Sisterhood
Peggy Brooks-Bertram

African sisters, we shook the universe last night
Our souls intermingled when we held on tight
to those whose voices cracked in pain
and those who thought they could abstain
with ancestors swirling all about and
urging us to sing and shout.
Demanding that we find the strength
to break the chains that cause
us African women pain.
Like men, and hair and shades of skin and
other demons locked within.
There were those who thought they could abstain
with ancestors swirling all about directing us to sing and shout.
"Raise your hands in her direction, give that
sister our protection."

Release her from this terrible pain, make this sister whole
again.
Demons begone!
Demons begone!
Demons begone!
African sisters with all our power demand you go
within the hour!
And still there were those who thought they could abstain with
ancestors swirling all about, urging us to sing and shout:
"This little light of mine, I'm gonna let it shine."
"This little light of mine, I'm gonna let it shine."
"This little light of mine, I'm gonna let it shine."
"Let it shine, let it shine, let it shine."
Someone hold that beautiful sister, soothe her fears,
kiss her face, wipe her tears.
One by one each in turn would find the strength
to stand and say,
I need you, I love you and I'm so glad
I'm here today.
'Til there were none who could abstain with
ancestors swirling all about directing
us to sing and shout, commanding
demons to come out!
We shook the universe last night!
Our souls intermingled as we held on tight and
promised each other to keep in touch
with the African sisterhood we need so much.

Copyright Peggy Brooks-Bertram, April 1990.

Selected Bibliography

Adkins, C. B. & Fields, J. (1992). Health care values of homeless women and their children. *Family Community Health,* 15 (3), 20–29.

AIDS in Black America: It's not just a gay thing. (1995). *Crisis,* 102 (5), 34–35.

Amaro, H., Beckman, L. J. & Mays, V. M. (1987). A comparison of black and white women entering alcoholism treatment. *Journal of Studies on Alcohol,* 43 (3), 220–228.

American Cancer Facts and Figures (1995). Atlanta: American Cancer Society, 95, 375 M-No. 5008.95.

Angelou, M. (1986). *All God's Children Need Traveling Shoes.* New York: Random House.

Angelou, M. (1969). *I Know Why The Caged Bird Sings.* New York: Random House.

Ashante, M. K. & Mattison, M. (1991). *Historical and Cultural Atlas of African-Americans.* New York: Macmillan.

Avery, B. Y. The health status of black women (1992). In R. Braithwaite & S. E. Taylor, eds., *Health Issues in the Black Community.* San Francisco: Jossey-Bass.

Barbee, E. (1994). Healing Time: The blues and African American women. *Health Care for Women International,* 15, 53–60.

Barbee, E. L. (1992). African American women and depression: A review and critique of the literature. *Archives of Psychiatric Nursing,* 7 (5), 257–265.

Bassuk, E. L. (1993). Social and economic hardships of homeless and other poor women. *American Journal Orthopsychiat,* 63 (3), 340–347.

Beale, Francis (1970). Double Jeopardy in the black woman. In Toni Cade, ed., *The Black Woman.* New York: Mentor/New American Library.

Beardsley, E. (1990). Race as a factor in health. In Rima Apple, ed., *Women, Health and Medicine in America: A Historical Handbook.* New York: Garland.

Billingsley, A. (1992). *Climbing Jacob's Ladder: The Enduring Legacy of African-American Families.* New York: Simon & Schuster.

Boring, C. C., Squires, T. S. & Heath, C. W. (1992). *Cancer Statistics for African Americans.* Atlanta: American Cancer Society, 92-20M-N-3034-PE.

Brent, L. (1973). *Incidents in the Life of a Slave Girl.* New York: Harcourt Brace Jovanovich.

Brown, D. & Gray, L. (1987). Social support and physical and mental health of urban black adults. *Journal of Human Stress,* Winter, 165–174.

Brown, D., Nilubuisi, S. & Gray, L. (1990). Religiosity and psychological distress among blacks. *Journal of Religion and Health,* 29, 55–68.

Brown, L. & Williams, R. D. (1994). Culturally sensitive breast cancer screening programs for older black women. *Nurse Practitioner,* 19 (3), 21–32.

Brown, M. L., Kessler, L. G. & Reuter, F. G. (1990). Is the supply of mammography machines outstripping need and demand? An economic analysis. *American International Medicine,* 113, 547–552.

Browne, A. (1993). Family violence and homelessness: The relevance of trauma histories in the lives of homeless women. *American Journal Orthopsychiat.,* 63 (3), 370–384.

Burack, Robert C. (1989). The acceptance and completion of mammography by older black women. *American Journal of Public Health,* 79, 721–726.

Caetano, R. (1984). Ethnicity and drinking in northern California: A comparison among whites, blacks, and hispanics. *Alcohol and Alcoholism,* 19, 31–44.

Caplan, L. S., Wells, B. L. & Haynes, S. (1992). Breast cancer screening among older racial/ethnic minorities and whites: Barriers to early detection. *Journal of Gerontology,* 47, 101–110.

Child Welfare League of America (1995). Multiethnic Placement Act of 1994, Briefing Paper. Washington, DC: CWLA.

Council Report. (1992). Induced termination of pregnancy before and after Roe v. Wade: Trends in the mortality and morbidity of women. *Journal of the American Medical Association,* 268 (22), 3231–3239.

Dalton, H. L. (1989). Aids in blackface. *Daedalus,* 118, 205–227.

Daniels, S. (1993). Women's health issues. In L. H. Talbott, E. Noble, & L. G. Klein, (eds.), *Women in the Heart of America: Concerns, Needs and Priority Issues for the 1990s.* The Women's Foundation of Greater Kansas City, MO.

Davis-Penn, D. (1992). Health Care Survey, Lincoln University, Department of Cooperative Extension and the Association for Gerontology and Human Development in Historically Black Colleges & Universities and Minority Management Interns for Missouri Department of Health.

Drayer, J. & Zegarelli, E. (1989). Hypertension and pregnancy. In P. Douglas, ed., *Heart Disease in Women.* Philadelphia: F. A. Davis Company.

Freund, P. & McGuire, M. (1991). *Health Issues and the Social Body: Critical Sociology*. Englewood Cliffs, NJ: Prentice Hall.

Giddings, P. (1984). *When and Where I Enter*. New York: Bantam Books.

Gray, S. & Nybell, L. (1990). Issues in African-American family preservation. *Child Welfare*, 69 (6), 513–523.

Hale, C. B. (1992). A demographic profile of African Americans. In R. Braithwaite and S. E. Taylor, eds., *Health Issues in the Black Community*. San Francisco: Jossey-Bass.

Hayes, P. (1993). Transracial adoption: politics and ideology. *Child Welfare*, 72 (3), 301–310.

Health Resources and Services Administration. (June 1994). Work Group on HIV/ AIDS Health Care Access Issues for African Americans. Rockville, MD.

Hildreth, C. & Saunders, E. (1991). Hypertension in Blacks: Clinical Overview. In Elijah Saunders, ed., *Cardiovascular Disease in Blacks*. Philadelphia: F. A. Davis Company.

Hogue, C. J. & Hargraves, M. A. (1993). Class, race and infant mortality in the U.S. *American Journal of Public Health*, 83 (1), 9–12.

hooks, bell. (1981). *Ain't I a Woman: Black Women and Feminism*. Boston: South End Press.

hooks, b. (1993). *Sisters of the Yam*. Boston: South End Press.

Horton, A. J. (ed.). (1992). *The Women's Health Data Book: A Profile of Women's Health in the United States*. Washington, DC: The Jacobs Institute of Women's Health.

Hudson-Weems, C. (1989). Cultural and agenda conflicts in academia: Critical issues for African women's studies. *Western Journal of Black Studies*, 13 (4), 185–189.

Hurston, Z. (1990). *Their Eyes Were Watching God*. New York: Harper & Row.

Jackson, M. (1993). Factors related to depression in African-American women. Unpublished Dissertation, University of Cincinnati.

Johnson, K. A. (1994). The color of health care. *Hearts and Soul*, Spring: 53–57.

Kalichman, S., Hunter, T. & Kelly, J. (1992). Perceptions of AIDS susceptability among minority and nonminority women at risk for HIV infection. *Journal of Counseling and Clinical Psychology*, 60, 725–732.

Kleinman, A. (1988). *The Illness Narrative: Suffering, Healing and the Human Condition*. New York: Basic Books.

Kost, K. & Forrest, J. D. (1995). Intention status of U.S. births in 1988: Differences by mothers' socioeconomic and demographic characteristics. *Family Planning Perspectives*, 27 (1), 11–17.

Land, H. (1994). Aids and women of color. *Families in Society: The Journal of Contemporary Human Services*, 6, 355–361.

Lee, F. R. & Gold, R. B. (1990). Empty womb: Black women's views on abortion. *Essence*, 21 (1), 51–52.

Leigh, W. (1994). *The Health Status of Women of Color*. A Women's Health Report of the Women's Research and Education Institute, Washington, DC.

Levine, C. D. & Dubler, N. (1990). Uncertain risks and bitter realities: The reproductive choices of HIV-infected women. *Milibank Quarterly*, 68 (3), 321.

Lillie-Blanton, M., MacKenzie, E. & Anthony, J. (1991). Black-white differences in alcohol use by women: Baltimore survey findings. *Public Health Reports,* 106 (2), 124–133.

Locke, D. (1992). *Increasing Multicultural Understanding.* Newbury Park, CA: Sage Publications.

Lorde, A. (1984). *Sister Outsider: Essays and Speeches by Audre Lorde.* Freedom, CA: The Crossing Press.

Lyons, J. (1972). Methods of successful communication with the disadvantaged. In *Communication for Change with the Rural Disadvantaged.* Washington, DC: National Academy of Sciences.

Mandela, N. (1994). *The Long Walk to Freedom.* London: Little, Brown.

McAdoo, H. (ed.). (1993). *Family Ethnicity.* Newbury Park, CA: Sage Publications.

McMillan, T. (1992). *Waiting to Exhale.* New York: Viking Press.

Mechanic, D. (1989). Socioeconomic status and health: An examination of underlying processes. In J. P. Bunker, D. S. Goinby & B. H. Kehrer, eds., *Pathways to Health: The Role of Social Factors.* Menlo Park, CA.: Henry J. Kaiser Foundation.

Mills, A. J. (1994). Systemic lupus erythematosus. *The New England Journal of Medicine,* 300 (26), 1871–1879.

Morrison, T. (1987). *Beloved.* New York: Alfred A. Knopf.

Morrison, T. (1973). *Sula.* New York: Alfred A. Knopf.

Myers, L. W. (1991). *Black Women Do they Cope Better?* San Francisco: Mellen Research University Press.

National Association of Black Social Workers. (1972). Position statement on transracial adoptions. Conference Proceedings, Nashville.

National Association of Black Social Workers. (1994). Position statement: Preserving African-American Families. Detroit: NABSW.

Nsiah-Jefferson, L. (1993). Access to reproductive genetic services for low income women and women of color. *Fetal Diagnosis Therapy,* 8, Supplement 1, 1-2-127.

O'Hara, W. P., Pollard, K. M., Mann, T. L. & Kent, M. M. (1991). African Americans in the 1990s. *Population Bulletin,* 46 (1), 2–40.

Ogunyemi, C. O. (1985). Womanism: The dynamics of the contemporary black female novel in English. *Signs: Journal of Women in Culture and Society,* 11 (1), 63–80.

Peterson, J. L., Catania, J. A., Dolcini, M. M. & Faigeles, B. (1993). Multiple sexual partners among blacks in high-risk cities. *Family Planning Perspectives,* 25 (6), 257–262.

Pinn, V. (1992). Women's health research: Prescribing change and addressing the issues. *Journal of The American Medical Association,* 268, 14.

Pohl, C. & Harris, W. (1992). *Transracial Adoption: Children and Parents Speak.* New York: Franklin Watts.

Price, J. H., Desmond, S. M., Slenker, S., Smith, D. & Stewart, P. W. (1992). Urban Black Woman's Perceptions of Breast Cancer and Mammography. *Journal of Community Health,* 17 (4), 191–204.

Reed, W. L., Darity, W. & Roberson, N. L. (1993). *Health and Medical Care of African Americans.* Westport, CT.: Auburn House.

Richie, B. (1994). AIDS: In living color. In E. White, ed., *Black Women's Health Book: Speaking for Ourselves.* Seattle: Seal Press.

Russell, K. & Jewell, N. (1992). Cultural impact of health-care access: Challenges for improving the health of African-Americans. *Journal of Community Health Nursing,* 9 (3), 161–169.

Saito, I., Takeshita, E., Hayashi, S. et al. (1990). Comparison of clinic and home blood pressure levels and the role of the sympathetic nervous system in clinic-home differences. *American Journal of Hypertension,* 3, 219.

Scott, K. Y. (1991). *The Habit of Surviving.* New York: Ballantine Books.

Scott-Jones, D. (1993). Adolescent childbearing: Whose problem? What can we do? *Phi Delta Kappan,* 75 (3), 1–12.

Silverman, A. (1993). Outcomes of transracial adoption. *The Future of Children,* 3 (1), 104–118.

Snapp, M. (1992). Occupational stress, social support, and depression among black and white professional-managerial women. *Women and Health,* 18 (1).

Spar, K. (1991). Child welfare and foster care reform: Issues for Congress. Washington, DC: Congressional Research Service, Library of Congress.

Stevenson, H. C. & Renard, G. (1993). Trusting ole' wise owls: Therapeutic use of cultural strengths in African-American families. *Professional Psychology: Research and Practice,* 24 (4), 433–442.

Stehlin, D. (1991). Living with lupus, DHHS Pub. No. (FDA)90-3178. A reprint from *FRD Consumer* magazine, December 1989–January 1990. U.S. Department of Health and Human Services, Public Health Services, Food and Drug Administration. Washington, DC: U.S. Government Printing Office.

Straussner, S. L. (1985). Alcoholism in women: Current knowledge and implications for treatment. *Alcoholism Treatment Quarterly,* 2 (1), 61–75.

Suchman, E. A. (1964). Sociomedical variations among ethnic groups. *American Journal of Sociology,* 70, 319–331.

U.S. Bureau of the Census. (1992). The black population in the United States, March 1991. *Current Population Reports,* Series P-20, No. 464. Washington, DC.: U.S. Government Printing Office.

U.S. Bureau of the Census. (1993). *We the American Blacks.* Washington, DC.: U.S. Government Printing Office.

Warren, B. J., Menke, E. M. & Clement, J. (1992). The mental health of African-American and Caucasian-American women who are homeless. *Journal of Psychosocial Nursing and Mental Health Services,* 30 (11), 27–30.

Washington, H. A. (1995). *Heart and Soul,* April.

Water, M. C. (1991). The role of lineage in identity formation among Black Americans. *Qualitative Social.,* 14 (1), 57–76.

Williams, D. H. (1986). The epidemiology of mental illness in Afro-Americans. *Hospital and Community Psychiatry,* 37 (1), 42–49.

Wilmore, G. (1973). *Black Religion and Black Radicalism.* Garden City, NY: Anchor Books.

Wilson, H. (1983). *Our Nig.* New York: Random House.

Wynne, M. J. (1985). Chitterlings, whiskey and colored folks: Chemical dependency in black Americans, an American dilemma. Unpublished manuscript.

Index

About the Editor and Contributors

CATHERINE FISHER COLLINS is Associate Professor at the State University of New York, Empire State College and Instructor at the State University of New York, Educational Opportunity Center. She is a Nurse Practitioner and certified in health education. She is the author of *Imprisoned African-American Women: Causes, Conditions and Future Implications* (1996).

PEGGY BROOKS-BERTRAM is the Executive Director of Jehudi Educational Services, a private woman-owned business that provides educational support and services to graduate students. She is also Executive Director of Bertram and Bertram Associates, a consulting firm specializing in disease management, quality assurance, case management, and health services research. Dr. Bertram also produces a local television program entitled "The Health Store."

CYNTHIA CRAWFORD-GREEN, MD is an Associate Professor at Howard University College of Medicine. She is also the director of the Nuclear Cardiology Laboratory at Howard University Hospital, serves as the Cardiology Fellowship Program Coordinator, and is actively involved in several funded research efforts. Her major research interests are myocardial ischemia, diabetes, and cardiovascular disease in women. She has a private practice at the university where she specializes in severe hypertension.

RENEÉ BOWMAN DANIEL is Associate Professor and Chairperson of the Department of Social Work and Sociology at Daemen College, Amherst, New York. She is a Certified Social Worker in New York State and is Chairperson for the Publications Committee, Association of Baccalaureate Social Work and Professional Advisory Board of the University of Buffalo Graduate School of Social Work.

STACEY DANIELS is Director of Research and Evaluation for the Ewing Marion Kauffman Foundation in Kansas City, Missouri, and also holds a faculty appointment as a Clinical Assistant Professor of Psychology at the University of Missouri-Kansas City School of Medicine. Her publications include book chapters and articles in the *Journal of Applied Psychology* and *Public Health Reports*.

DOLORES DAVIS-PENN is the State Gerontology Specialist at Lincoln University Cooperative Extension in Jefferson City, Missouri. From 1992 to the present she has been the coordinator for the National Cancer Institutes Missouri National Black Leadership Initiative Rural Intervention and Evaluation Project, and is also the project director for the Missouri Department of Health's Breast and Cervical Cancer Control Project.

IMANI LILLIE B. FRYAR is a womanist who directs the Transitional Program at SUNY Empire State College. She is adjunct professor at SUNY Buffalo's African American Studies Department; at Rochester's Colgate Seminary where she teaches the Bible as Literature; at the National Congress of Christian Education, where she teaches Creative Teaching Methods, Motivating Adults and African American History; and is a consultant for American College Testing.

JUANITA K. HUNTER is a Clinical Associate Professor in the School of Nursing at the University of Buffalo, New York. She teaches in the undergraduate program with emphasis on community health, health care of vulnerable populations, and poverty. She served as project director of the Nursing Center for the Homeless, a program funded by the U.S. Department of Health and Human Services, from 1987 to 1993.

JACQUELINE D. SKILLERN JACKSON is in private practice in Palo Alto, California, and lecturer in the Alcohol Studies Program at the University of California.

BARBARA A. SEALS NEVERGOLD is the Executive Director of Planned Parenthood of Buffalo and Erie County, Inc. and Adjunct Professor at the State University of New York, Empire State College. She formerly was Executive Director of Foster Care Services in Neighborhood House, Lackawanna, NY. Her major emphasis for the past two years has been in the development of peer education programs, assuring continuity of care and catapulting the agency into the managed care arena as well as expanding the agency's participation into primary care.

NOMA L. ROBERSON is Director of Community Intervention and Research, Department of Cancer Control and Epidemiology at Roswell Park Cancer Institute in Buffalo, New York. She also is Program Evaluator with the University of Vermont Office of Health Promotion Research, College of Medicine in Burlington; and is the administrator for a Mobile Screening and Evaluation Clinic, which provides health services to women in several Western New York Counties.

E. GINGER SULLIVAN is a political scientist, lawyer, health advocate, researcher, physical therapist, and the founding president of Sullivan Transitions in Atlanta, Georgia.

ISBN 0-86569-250-5

EAN

9 780865 692503

HARDCOVER BAR CODE